Aligner Systems in Invisible Orthodontics

Stefan Abela

Aligner Systems in Invisible Orthodontics

Basic Concepts and Clinical Management

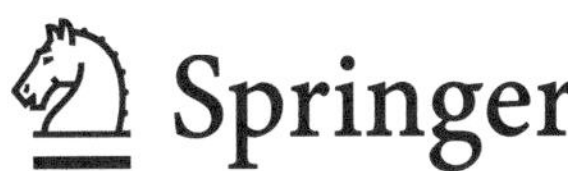 Springer

Stefan Abela
Cambridge, UK

ISBN 978-3-031-49206-8   ISBN 978-3-031-49204-4   (eBook)
https://doi.org/10.1007/978-3-031-49204-4

This Springer imprint is published by the registered company Springer Nature Switzerland AG
The registered company address is: Gewerbestrasse 11, 6330 Cham, Switzerland

Paper in this product is recyclable.

Preface

This book provides the reader with an in-depth knowledge of the processes involved in providing aligner treatment and describes the techniques and biomechanics involved in providing orthodontic treatment solely with aligners or in combination with other types of appliances.

There has been, over the years, various opinions and contention with regard to the adequacy of providing orthodontic treatment with aligners. Some cases would certainly benefit from this technique in contrast to others that will be worse off in comparison to being treated with other techniques still considered to be the gold standard within the specialty.

Evidence supporting the clear aligner technique remains sparse; however, more studies are being carried out to prove the aligners' clinical abilities and compare them to more traditional techniques principally involving removable and fixed appliances.

Although a vast range of aligner manufacturers and types are available in the market, and this book is completely unbiased, Invisalign® by Align Technology, Inc., remains the market leader and the one most widely used by clinicians at an international level. Consequently, this position has been respected by the author and its usage was reflected during the composition and collation of the latest available information and scientific evidence for this book.

This book, innovative in nature, will provide the reader with an invaluable depth of knowledge with regard to the various types of aligners, the techniques used in their application, the practical aspects of delivery and the scientific data available to back their everyday use.

Cambridge, UK

Stefan Abela

September 2023

Acknowledgements

This book is dedicated to my wife, Dr Milisha Chotai for her infinite help and support in seeing me through completion of this textbook which needed intense preparation, research and analysing completed clinical cases leaving me with no time on many occasions to dedicate to my family.

Introduction

The increased demand for discreet orthodontic treatment is a widely perceived and accepted phenomenon, and this increased demand has been further exacerbated with the introduction of aligners. With the increased popularity of aligner systems, the number of adults seeking orthodontic treatment has similarly increased exponentially [1, 2]. The superiority over other orthodontic systems include the following:

– Aesthetic discreetness [3]
– Risk reduction of periodontal complications during active treatment [4]
– Comfort and adaptability [5]
– Freedom over masticatory choice [6, 7]
– Possibility of monitoring the progress of treatment remotely [8]
– Provision of efficient mechanics and satisfactory outcomes [9]
– Reduction in operator chair-side time [1, 10]
– Possibility of usage in conjunction with other orthodontic auxiliaries [11]

The current international aligner market is worth around 2 billion USD (US Dollar), but consumer data reports estimate a four-fold market increase by 2028. Reports by Statista, Inc., Ströer Content Group, GmbH, Hamburg, Germany, and by ©Grand View Research, Inc., Los Angeles, USA, are in agreement whilst reports by MarketStudyReport, Pune, India, have forecasted a year-on-year growth between 2021 and 2027 of 27 % leading to a global market value of 14 billion USD in value. The global oral care value is estimated to be around 55 billion USD by 2025, so one cannot leave the proportion dedicated to improving smile aesthetics unnoticed.

Analysis of web searching trends as a reflection of future patients' choices will also increase with a study suggesting an increase of a minimum of 6 % to a maximum of 13 % with the analysis extending to three European countries. This was drawn in direct comparison to the previous year (2021) [12].

On balance, although Align Technology, Inc., California, USA, might be viewed as the most popular aligner manufacturer, other leading aligner systems include: ClearCorrect by Straumann Group Basel, Switzerland;, Spark by Ormco™, California, USA; SureSmile® Dentsply North Carolina, USA; 3M™ Clarity Aligners, 3M Minnesota, USA; F22 Aligner by Sweden & Martina, Padua, Italy; Nuvola® Clear Aligners by GEO Srl, Vicenza, Italy; CA® Clear Aligners by Scheu-Dental GmbH, Iserlohn, Germany; iROK™ Aligners by iROK™ Digital Dental

Studio, California, USA; Angelalign by Angelalign Technology, Inc., Shanghai, China; Alineadent Aligners by Alineadent, Malaga, Spain; Orthocaps TwinAligner® System by Rocky Mountains, Indiana, USA; K Clear and Clear X by K Line, Düsseldorf-Benrath, Germany; EZ-X by DynaFlex®, Missouri, USA; eXceed aligners, by eXceed®, Witten, Germany; Accusmile® by Forestadent, Pforzheim, Germany; smart moves® by Great Lakes Dental Technologies, New York, USA; SLX™ Clear Aligner System and Reveal® by Henry Schein, New York, USA; Refine® by TP Orthodontics, Indiana, USA.

Direct consumer companies, most notably Smile Direct Club™ LLC, Tennessee, USA, aim at providing a direct aligner provision to the customers avoiding the doctor to patient interaction enabling direct entry into the market at a much lower price bracket. Other remotely monitoring aligner systems include Candid™ Aligners, New York, USA; NewSmile™ Aligners, Vancouver, British Columbia, and Byte® Aligners, California, USA, and AlignerCo, New York, USA. Emergence of new providers and cessation of existing ones is a continuously fluid model due to the related costs of production, shipping, marketing and other related costs. In-house production of aligners could also provide a challenge with increasingly user-friendly software and 3D printing facilities becoming more financially accessible.

Most of the scientific articles directly related to orthodontic aligners have been published in the last 10 to 20 years. This trend is also expected to increase as the technique becomes more widespread and clinical advances using this technique together with any accompanying auxiliaries, accomplished.

Clear aligners have seen a significant improvement in their accompanying attachments' design that play a key role with expressing the desired tooth movement [13]. The aligners' flexibility of being used with other appliances further expands their scope rendering their use in orthognathic cases very feasible [11].

The biomaterials, mainly in the form of thermoplastic polymers have also seen an improvement in their physical and mechanical properties and have been extensively researched [14, 15]. The thermoforming process normally takes place on an accurate representation of a patient's dental models and although at this early stage, the materials undergo a change in their properties, their clinical use is not compromised. Further changes to their properties are mediated with the exposure of the intraoral environment. Changes in the their physical composition are rendered tangible with the continuous exposure of moisture, elevated temperatures in comparison to room temperature, elastic deformation and increased stiffness with alterations to their crystalline morphological composition [16, 17]. This phenomenon has led to aligner manufacturers recommending a time interval between successive stages, i.e. between 7 and 14 days.

A key factor to the behaviour and characteristics of an aligner is the thickness used to manufacture it. In general, the thickness of aligners varies between 0.5 mm and 1 mm. The manufacturing process might also bear an influence on the final aligner thickness [18]. The thickness has a directly proportional relationship with the delivery of the orthodontic forces needed for tooth movement but also with the amount of ageing exhibited with intraoral use over time [19].

The future, as alluded to above, will not only see an increase and an improvement with the current techniques but also will progress to incorporate more complex digitisation processes. This will include incorporation of Cone-Beam Computed Tomography (CBCT) data to enable better prediction of crown-root movements and enable full customisation of the appliances, better integration with enhanced software systems to facilitate in-house production by individual clinicians and an increase in both industrial-scale production and direct home delivery systems.

The recently adopted technologies have helped propel aligners to an everyday proposition amongst both general dental practitioners and specialist practitioners. Technologies involving 3D printing, CAD-CAM, and thermoprocessing allowed this uptake and widespread acceptance. The next generation of aligners will adopt four-dimensional (4D) properties with the introduction of the shape memory polymers (SMPs). These new materials will possess the ability to allow changes to the aligners' shape during intraoral use to improve efficacy to yet another level [20].

Another prospective developmental advancement in aligner therapy could be in an extremely rapid turnaround time for production and delivery rendering same-day finalisation of the product very realistic, especially when considering the gigantic advancements in CAT technology. This leap could be potentially attained by the elimination of 3D model printing and thermoforming processes altogether.

The individual manufacturers claim unique selling points and advantageous characteristics over their competitors. These claims are hard to identify; however, the clinician remains solely responsible for ensuring the treatment efficacy and safety of the patient undergoing treatment. Precautions, such as optimal communication and clear outlining of expectations, will ensure successful outcomes. In the case of orthodontic aligners specifically, thorough treatment planning and an immeasurable knowledge of the planning software together with setting realistic tooth movement goals will be key in allowing the clinician to relay the results from a digital platform to a realistic dimension.

References

1. Tamer I, Oztas E, Marsan G. Orthodontic treatment with clear aligners and the scientific reality behind their marketing: a literature review. Turk J Orthod. 2019;32(4):241–6.
2. Macrì MMG, Varvara G, Traini T, Festa F. Clinical performances and biological features of clear aligners materials in orthodontics. Front Mater. 2022;9:1–10.
3. Bucci R, Rongo R, Levate C, Michelotti A, Barone S, Razionale AV, et al. Thickness of orthodontic clear aligners after thermoforming and after 10 days of intraoral exposure: a prospective clinical study. Prog Orthod. 2019;20(1):36.
4. Miethke RR, Brauner K. A comparison of the periodontal health of patients during treatment with the Invisalign system and with fixed lingual appliances. J Orofac Orthop. 2007;68(3):223–31.
5. White DW, Julien KC, Jacob H, Campbell PM, Buschang PH. Discomfort associated with Invisalign and traditional brackets: a randomized, prospective trial. Angle Orthod. 2017;87(6):801–8.

6. Flores-Mir C, Brandelli J, Pacheco-Pereira C. Patient satisfaction and quality of life status after 2 treatment modalities: Invisalign and conventional fixed appliances. Am J Orthod Dentofacial Orthop. 2018;154(5):639–44.

7. Zhang B, Huang X, Huo S, Zhang C, Zhao S, Cen X, et al. Effect of clear aligners on oral health-related quality of life: a systematic review. Orthod Craniofac Res. 2020;23(4):363–70.

8. Sangalli L, Savoldi F, Dalessandri D, Bonetti S, Gu M, Signoroni A, et al. Effects of remote digital monitoring on oral hygiene of orthodontic patients: a prospective study. BMC Oral Health. 2021;21(1):435.

9. Rossini G, Parrini S, Castroflorio T, Deregibus A, Debernardi CL. Efficacy of clear aligners in controlling orthodontic tooth movement: a systematic review. Angle Orthod. 2015;85(5):881–9.

10. Zheng M, Liu R, Ni Z, Yu Z. Efficiency, effectiveness and treatment stability of clear aligners: a systematic review and meta-analysis. Orthod Craniofac Res. 2017;20(3):127–33.

11. Kankam HKN, Gupta H, Sawh-Martinez R, Steinbacher DM. Segmental multiple-jaw surgery without orthodontia: clear aligners alone. Plast Reconstr Surg. 2018;142(1):181–4.

12. Sycinska-Dziarnowska M, Szyszka-Sommerfeld L, Wozniak K, Lindauer SJ, Spagnuolo G. Predicting interest in orthodontic aligners: a google trends data analysis. Int J Environ Res Public Health. 2022;19(5):3105.

13. Dasy H, Dasy A, Asatrian G, Rozsa N, Lee HF, Kwak JH. Effects of variable attachment shapes and aligner material on aligner retention. Angle Orthod. 2015;85(6):934–40.

14. Lombardo L, Arreghini A, Bratti E, Mollica F, Spedicato G, Merlin M, et al. Comparative analysis of real and ideal wire-slot play in square and rectangular archwires. Angle Orthod. 2015;85(5):848–58.

15. Liu CL, Sun WT, Liao W, Lu WX, Li QW, Jeong Y, et al. Colour stabilities of three types of orthodontic clear aligners exposed to staining agents. Int J Oral Sci. 2016;8(4):246–53.

16. Eliades T, Bourauel C. Intraoral aging of orthodontic materials: the picture we miss and its clinical relevance. Am J Orthod Dentofacial Orthop. 2005;127(4):403–12.

17. Alexandropoulos A, Al Jabbari YS, Zinelis S, Eliades T. Chemical and mechanical characteristics of contemporary thermoplastic orthodontic materials. Aust Orthod J. 2015;31(2):165–70.

18. Edelmann A, English JD, Chen SJ, Kasper FK. Analysis of the thickness of 3-dimensional-printed orthodontic aligners. Am J Orthod Dentofacial Orthop. 2020;158(5):e91–e8.

19. Ren C, Li X, Wang Z, Wang H, Bai Y. Measurement of orthodontic forces exerted on the upper right central incisor with the increase of the distance of tooth movement and thickness of the aligner. Zhonghua Kou Qiang Yi Xue Za Zhi. 2014;49(3):177–9.

20. Elshazly TM, Keilig L, Alkabani Y, Ghoneima A, Abuzayda M, Talaat W, Talaat S, Bourauel C. Potential application of 4D technology in fabrication of orthodontic aligners. Front Mater. 2022;8:794536.

Contents

Part IV   Technological Apps to Aid Aligner Therapy

Part V   Evidence-Based Aligner Therapy

About the Author

Stefan Abela, BChD, MFDS, MSc, MOrth Dr Stefan Abela is a Specialist, a distinguised Consultant in Orthodontics, directing private practices in London and in Ely, Cambridgeshire within the United Kingdom and an internationally renowned speaker. He obtained his first qualification from the Malta Medical School, University of Malta, Msida, Malta in 2003. To date, he has obtained numerous postgraduate qualifications from The Royal College of Surgeons of England and Edinburgh including a full membership and fellowship with consistent standout contributions to the international scientific community and to the profession. He has been actively involved in the UK's national education and training programme of postgraudate trainees and has been a former head of department at the Norfolk and Norwich University Hospital NHS Foundation Trust, Norwich, UK. Considered an international leader within the profession, he is an avid academic contributor and continuously publishes scientific articles in the highest ranking internationally peer-reviewed journals. He is also an internationally best-selling author of medical text-books with his previous textbook entitled *Leadership and Management in Healthcare: A Guide for Medical and Dental Practitioners.*

Abbreviations

ABO	American Board of Orthodontics
AI	Artificial Intelligence
A-P	Antero-posterior
BPR	Buccal power ridges
BSSO	Bilateral sagittal split osteotomy
CAD	Computer-aided design
CAM	Computer-aided manufacturing
CBCT	Cone-beam computed tomography
GCF	Gingival crevicular fluid
ICP	Intercuspal position
IDS	Invisalign Doctor Site
IMF	Intermaxillary fixation
IOSim	Invisalign® Outcome Simulator
IPR	Interproximal reduction
LL	Lower left
LR	Lower right
LRT	Lingual root torque
MM	Millimetre
OB	Overbite
OJ	Overjet
OMI	Orthodontic mini-implant
PC	Polycarbonate
PET	Polyethylene terephthalate
PETG	Polyethylene terephthalate glycol
PI	Plaque index
PP	Polypropylene
PVS	Polyvinylsiloxane
RCT	Randomised controlled trial
SM	Study model
SMP	Shape memory polymers
STL	Standard triangle language
TMJD	Temporomandibular joint dysfunction
TPU	Thermoplastic polyurethane
UL	Upper left

UR	Upper right
VCC	Virtual C-Chain
VPC	Virtual power chain
WM	Working model

Part I

Basic Concepts and Materials

General Aligner Concepts

1

1.1   Introduction

Aligner treatment is very different to more widely used appliances such as fixed appliances. The biomechanics are consequentially very different too. This chapter aims at highlighting these differences and also gives an insight into the development of Invisalign® and its various iterations by evolving with each progressive generation. This chapter will also describe the process of force generation by aligners and how these forces are selectively transferred onto the surfaces of the teeth effectively with the ultimate aim being that of delivering a very efficient system to both the treating clinician and the end user, the patient.

Align Technology, Inc., albeit being the main and leading market provider of aligners, an uncountable number of companies are currently producing aligners with claims that they all have different features and provide added value to the clinicians' clients. In-house manufacturing of aligners is also currently commonplace with readily available digital intraoral scanners and software packages allowing the clinician to directly relay the prescription to the software and 3D printers, making small-scale production of aligners very feasible. A more contemporary approach to obtain a segment of this market is the direct consumer approach taken by several companies, also referred to as home aligners companies.

1.2   Developmental Stages of Invisalign®

The first stage of the development process came about with the use of PC30, Proceed30, the preferred polymer at the time, back in 1999. One of the first reported uses of Invisalign® aligners for space closure and relief of mildly crowded cases was available shortly afterwards in 2001 [1]. PC30 had both physical and chemical limitations which in turn limited the range of orthodontic cases that aligners could be used for [2].

© The Author(s), under exclusive license to Springer Nature Switzerland AG 2024
S. Abela, *Aligner Systems in Invisible Orthodontics*,
https://doi.org/10.1007/978-3-031-49204-4_1

Within 8 years, in 2009, the second generation of aligners by Align Technology, Inc. was available featuring the inclusion of attachments to render specific tooth movements more easily. These were called SmartForce® features aimed at addressing vertical and rotatory movements of teeth.

The third generation (G3) followed the year after in 2010 offering the user the possibility of inserting precision cuts for the use of inter arch elastics. G3 has also allowed the introduction of lingual root torque (LRT).

G4 or the fourth generation followed closely in 2011 with the aim of improving the management of anterior open bites and root tip control. Further improvements were seen in 2013 with the use of SmartTrack® for improved control of tooth movements by increasing the efficacy of tooth to material interface. G5, introduced the year after, in 2014 allowed deep bite correction improvements, deemed a feature of malocclusion that aligners were not on par with conventional appliances. Bite ramps, an added feature on the palatal aspect of the upper incisors, were designed to mimic the effect of anterior bite planes used in conventional appliances.

The launch of G6 ensued in 2015 with the aim of improving anchorage control for extraction cases. The seventh generation, G7 launched in 2016, decreased aligner time to 1 week at a time decreasing treatment duration and introduced molar attachments to minimise posterior open bites due to buccal segments disocclusion. In 2017, Invisalign Teen® expanded the scope of use of aligners to a younger age group making allowances for the various mixed dentition stages.

Prior to the launch of the current generation, G8 introduced in 2020, Invisalign Go and Invisalign First were also introduced by Align Technology, Inc. The former provided a chair-side platform for general dental practitioners whilst Invisalign First allowed an initial phase for younger patients acting as an interceptive phase that is known to take place in more conventional orthodontic pathways prior to the definitive fixed appliance phase for the final correction of the malocclusion. The G8 expanded the scope of aligners once more providing correction possibilities for crossbites and more severe cases of dental crowding. In 2021 and 2022, further advancements and improvements to ClinCheck® Pro 6.0 software were witnessed by the users. These included:

1. "In-face" visualisation to preempt the facial changes visually following Invisalign treatment.
2. CBCT integration to enable 3D visualisation of the patients' dentoalveolar complex including roots, crowns, and alveolar bone.

1.3 G8

Invisalign latest generation, the eighth, referred to G8 remains the most contemporary version of aligner from Align Technology, Inc., San Jose, California, USA.

G8 utilises SmartForce® activation to enable specific areas within the aligner surfaces to act on specific areas of a tooth to bring about more efficient and targeted tooth movements. These innovations that pertain to G8 will have been applied to all the aligners fabricated prospectively from 2021. Certain features of SmartForce®

are automatically triggered by ClinCheck® Pro 6.0, and the priority hierarchy for the G8 protocol is pre-set by the software's algorithm.

The hierarchy prioritisation is in the order listed below:

1. Premolar extraction and multi-tooth extrusion movements
2. Optimised expansion support
3. Root movements
4. Single tooth movements including vertical and de-rotations
5. Anchorage for intrusion
6. Power ridge for adequate lingual root torque (LRT)

The acclaimed advantages over the previous generations are mainly two:

 (i) Improved ability to manage deep bites
(ii) Improved ability to manage crossbites involving the upper arch

1.3.1   Deep Bite Management with the Eighth Generation

The features introduced to G8 that were designed to manage deep bites more effectively include the following:

– Automatic software addition of bite ramps on the palatal aspect of the upper incisors when vertical correction is equal or greater than 1.5 mm.
– Overcorrection of lower incisor intrusion to flatten the curve of Spee. This is automatically incorporated by the software's algorithm.
– Optimised attachments to the lower lateral incisors with a dome-shaped design to provide vertical anchorage for neighbouring incisors when vertical discrepancies are present in the lower labial segment. The threshold for this discrepancy is when the vertical discrepancy is equal to or greater than 1 mm.
– En-masse intrusion to provide optimised intrusion on each individual incisor tooth. This is even more relevant if the initial position of the incisors differ vertically.

1.3.2   CrossBite Management with the Eighth Generation

The features introduced to G8 that were designed to manage crossbites more effectively by posterior arch expansion include the following:

– Individual posterior expansion forces for a more balanced expansion within the buccal segments and within the arch.
– Automatic placement of buccal root torque to avoid a consequential tip of palatal cusps and a reduction in overbite and less than ideal palatal cusp to lower occlusal surface contact.

- Optimised horizontal dome-shaped attachments on premolars and first molars with a de-rotatory movement which is invariably needed especially to the mesial aspect of the first molars.
- Prioritisation of expansion as the second most important movement with a threshold level of 0.5 mm.

1.4 ClinCheck® Pro 6.0

This proprietary software by Align Technology, Inc., San Jose, California, USA, is a cloud-based system that allows the capturing of a patient's virtual arches separately or in occlusion. The software is accessible by clinicians only; however, it is beneficial for both patients and clinicians. For the former, the visualisation of their occlusion at the start and the simulation of the treatment effects makes it easier to follow the tooth movements required to obtain the desired outcome. For the latter, the online 3D rendition can be used for visualisation purposes too, edited to improve outcomes, and usage as a monitoring tool to follow their progress. Both clinicians and clinical staff have access to the tools that the software provides to permit the greatest potential of tooth movement for the patient.

The latest innovations that have been introduced to the software include the following:

- Live or real-life updates to the corrections submitted on the Invisalign Doctor Site (IDS)
- CBCT integration to allow user manipulation of both the coronal and radicular aspects of the teeth
- "In-Face visualisation" that portrays the facial effects with the end result following treatment

1.4.1 ClinCheck® Pro 6.0 3D Features

The features available for the clinical team are available on the IDS (Invisalign Doctor Site) once the logging process has been completed.

Figure 1.1 below illustrates the second bar on the IDS with all the features at the disposition of the clinicians.

The icons representing the various features on the IDS represent different visualisation modes, diagnostics or tools to enhance the patients' outcomes. The features included in the treatment plan are represented with a blue dot next to the icon whilst those visible on the IDS platform are represented by a blue line under the

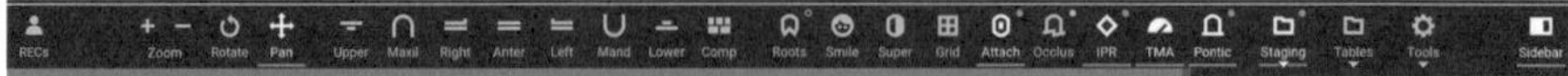

Fig. 1.1 The second bar on the IDS depicting all the 3D features available for the user. This diagram has been obtained from the ClinCheck Pro 6® software and reproduced by kind permission of Align Technology, Inc. (San Jose, California, USA)

icon. Starting from the far left, for visualisation purposes, the user has the following features listed below as they appear on the IDS from the left side.

1. "Zoom + or Zoom −" allows the user to magnify or minimise the view.
2. "Rotate" function allows the user to rotate the 3D virtual models.
3. "Pan" function to shift the position of the virtual models within the screen to allow the user to magnify an area of interest.
4. "Upper" allows the user to view the frontal aspect of the maxilla in isolation.
5. "Maxil" allows the user to view the occlusal aspect of the maxilla in isolation.
6. "Right" allows the user to view the right-hand side of the 3D models.
7. "Anterior" provides the user with a frontal view of the 3D models.
8. "Left" allows the user to view the left-hand side of the 3D models.
9. "Mand" allows the user to view the occlusal aspect of the mandible in isolation.
10. "Lower" allows the user to view the occlusal aspect of the mandible in isolation.
11. "Comp" short for composite view which allows the user to visualise five aspects of the 3D models: frontal, right, left, maxillary and mandibular occlusal views.
12. "Roots" allows the user to visualise the position of roots, bone and unerupted teeth.
13. "Smile" allows visualisation of the patient's postoperative results in the facial mailing extraoral photo.
14. "Super" short for superimposition visualises the original position of the teeth in comparison to the predicted end result. The original tooth position is coloured on the IDS.
15. "Grid" allows the user to have the 3D virtual models against a gridded background where each pixel of the grit is equivalent to 1 mm.
16. "Attach" allows the user to visualise the use of attachments, precision cuts, bite ramps and other auxiliary features included in the treatment plan.
17. "Occlus" allows the user to visualise the degree of inter arch contact points. Upon activation, the 3D models are rendered translucent to visualise the contact points better. A red dot next to the "Occlus" icon represents heavy contact points whilst green shows normal occlusal contact points. The red and green colours are used on the occlusal surfaces of the 3D models and equally represent the degree of inter arch occlusal contact points.
18. "IPR" represents interproximal reduction showing the amount of IPR prescribed by the clinician. This icon also represents any residual spacing present in the predicted outcome.
19. "TMA" represents tooth movement assessment and allows the user to verify the tooth movements incorporated to generate the end result on the ClinCheck®.
20. "Pontic" allows the user to activate the visualisation of any Pontics in sites where teeth are missing, unerupted or impacted.
21. "Stages" tab activation allows the user to:
    (i) Visualise the stage of specific tooth movements in their ClinCheck® simulation via the "Staging Panel"
    (ii) Visualise the bite corrections via the "Bite correction visualisation"
    (iii) Visualise any overcorrective tooth movements via the "Overcorrection" tab

22. "Tables" which allows the user to access the "Tooth movements table," the "Bolton Analysis," the "Arch width table," the "Overjet and overbite table" and the "Tooth numbering." Further details about tooth-size discrepancies can be found in Sect. 6.4.2.
23. "Tools" allows the user to access the "Eruption compensation" and "Occlusal plan inclination."

The "Sidebar" can be activated on the right-hand side of the IDS and allows the user to visualise previously agreed ClinCheck plans and instructions given to the Align Technology, Inc. technicians.

1.5   Space Closure Using Aligners

The indications for space closure with aligners as with other type of orthodontic appliances are brought about with increasingly difficult occlusions to manage. This is certainly the case when crowding is assessed as moderate or severe with over 6 mm of crowding in one or both arches and when the occlusion demands an extraction approach [3].

Classically, in orthodontics cases that need to be treated on an extraction basis require first or second premolar extractions. This renders the treatment more complex independent of the type of appliances used; however, the complexity of tooth control is even higher with clear aligner therapy. The main challenge is to control the tipping of the teeth adjacent to the extraction site with some authors suggesting a combination approach involving both clear aligners and fixed appliances [4].

Space closure and space management can be managed in one of the three ways listed below:

1. Predominant labial segment retraction.
2. Predominant buccal segment protraction.
3. A combination of the above.

Using clear aligners to retract incisors poses two main problems to the clinician:

(a) Torque loss in the labial segments.
(b) Exhibition of the bowing phenomenon.

In fixed appliance therapy, although the clinician can face the same clinical challenges, a selection of different archwires with varying degrees of stiffness enabling space closure without biomechanical sequelae are available. With clear aligner therapy, the flexibility inherent in the materials used to manufacture clear aligners will lead to unwanted movements as follows:

– Anteriorly, a clockwise movement with extrusion and relative increase in overbite leading to premature contacts with torque loss of the incisors.

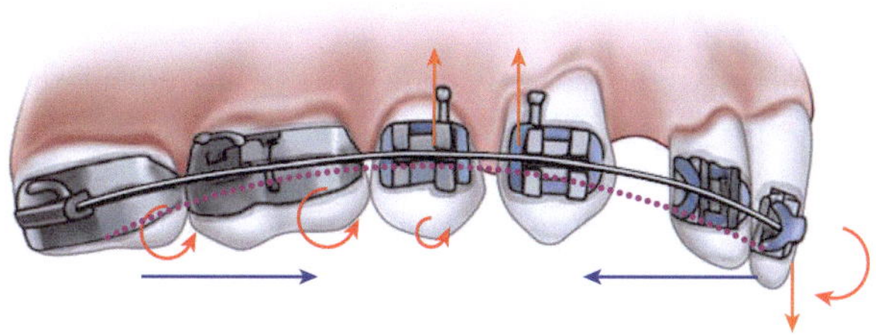

Fig. 1.2 Illustrates the "bowing" effect that could be seen during space closure during aligner therapy

- Posteriorly, an anticlockwise movement of the molars.
- Mid-arch in the premolar section, vertical intrusion is apparent earlier on in the space closure phase leading to a mid-arch open bite.

This phenomenon described above is known as "bowing" and is illustrated in Fig. 1.2 below.

Overcoming and minimising the bowing effects in clear aligner therapy warrants the following:

1. Additional anchorage reinforcement with the use of:
   (a) Inter arch elastics.
   (b) Orthodontic mini-implants.
2. Controlling the amount of tooth movement found in each tray. This can be done by either:
   (a) Minimising the quantity of space closure prescribed in each tray.
   (b) Alternating the treatment stages between active and passive aligners.
   (c) Alternating between space closure and specific tooth movements in the anterior or posterior segments.
   (d) Prescribe specific distalisation movements for the upper canines between space closure stages. This will decrease the risk of torque loss to the upper incisors and relative extrusion, maintaining overall control of the incisor inclination.
3. Introduction of a positive curve of Spee in the upper arch to counteract the negative sequelae described above.
4. Prescription of antagonistic tooth movements in the space closure phases such as extrusion of premolars, proclination of upper incisor crowns, intrusion of incisors and distal tipping of the molar crowns.
5. Strategic use of attachments that provide more vertical control of the incisors, premolars and molars, bilaterally. The attachments could be used for both active and retentive purposes such as optimised extrusive attachments and optimised retention attachments, respectively.
6. Use of vertical inter arch elastics in the premolar section using buttons to allow more efficient extrusive movements.

1.6   Mode of Action of Aligners

The clear Aligners' mechanism of tooth movement revolves around two main types:

1. Displacement-driven system.
2. Force-driven system [5, 6].

1.6.1 Displacement-Driven System

Aligners relying on a displacement-driven system need to have the sequential tooth movements staged and the aligners produced for each stage with the respective tooth movements in-built within each individual tray. The movement is solely based on the individual aligners' shape and once the aligner actuates the movements for each stage, it is rendered passive.

This process entails a more laborious and time-consuming approach with limited control of root movements. The obtainable movements for this type of system are primarily tipping and mild de-rotatory movements.

1.6.2 Force-Driven System

With aligner systems utilising this mode of action, the tooth movement predictions are mainly accomplished with CAD-CAM systems. Algorithms play a main role and are the main driver determining the sequential tooth movements. Placement of attachments and the stages are also based on algorithmic calculations. Biomechanically, tooth movements with these types of aligners are produced by changing the shape of the aligners at every stage. Obtaining a close adaptation of the aligner to each individual tooth surface creates strategic pressure points on the surfaces in addition to those generated by the presence of attachments. Other auxiliary features such as power ridges may also enhance tooth movement.

References

1. Vlaskalic V, Boyd R. Orthodontic treatment of a mildly crowded malocclusion using the Invisalign system. Aust Orthod J. 2001;17(1):41–6.
2. Phan X, Ling PH. Clinical limitations of Invisalign. J Can Dent Assoc. 2007;73(3):263–6.
3. Duncan LO, Piedade L, Lekic M, Cunha RS, Wiltshire WA. Changes in mandibular incisor position and arch form resulting from Invisalign correction of the crowded dentition treated nonextraction. Angle Orthod. 2016;86(4):577–83.
4. Baldwin DK, King G, Ramsay DS, Huang G, Bollen AM. Activation time and material stiffness of sequential removable orthodontic appliances. Part 3: premolar extraction patients. Am J Orthod Dentofacial Orthop. 2008;133(6):837–45.
5. Tamer I, Oztas E, Marsan G. Orthodontic treatment with clear aligners and the scientific reality behind their marketing: a literature review. Turk J Orthod. 2019;32(4):241–6.
6. Drake CT, McGorray SP, Dolce C, Nair M, Wheeler TT. Orthodontic tooth movement with clear aligners. ISRN Dent. 2012;2012:657973.

Types of Aligner Systems Available

2

2.1   Introduction

The increased uptake of clear aligner therapy has certainly been multifactorial. The CAD-CAM technology has rendered the delivery of aligners very tangible and eased production whilst social media and the search for more discreet solutions has fuelled this uptake further especially in adults.

In practice, there are three main types of aligners as follows:

1. Aligners manufactured by a certified company involving a doctor-to-patient interface
2. Direct-to-consumer aligners distributed directly to the patient
3. In-house manufacturing by the treatment provider

Public availability of direct-to-consumer aligners has raised concerns due to potential clinical risks of unsupervised treatment. The most notable ones amongst others are listed below:

1. Lack of caries detection
2. Development of working and non-working side interferences
3. Root resorption
4. Instability of periodontal disease
5. Loss of vitality monitoring

It is indisputable that clear aligners are more convenient and are a much more attractive orthodontic solution to patients. This is equally valid for both adults and teenagers with a better overall experience when compared to other types of orthodontic appliances. Studies have reported a lower impact on the quality of life during treatment with clear aligners when compared to fixed appliances [1]. Similarly, clear aligner therapy resulted in better pain perception by patients and overall satisfaction levels [2].

© The Author(s), under exclusive license to Springer Nature Switzerland AG 2024
S. Abela, *Aligner Systems in Invisible Orthodontics*,
https://doi.org/10.1007/978-3-031-49204-4_2

Despite the above-mentioned positive outcomes and a better perceived outlook by patients, aligner treatment does not have the same scientific backing as other appliances. Despite being in the market for over 20 years, evidence remains sparse and of low levels. There are certainly disagreements amongst clinicians as to what type of malocclusions aligners can be successfully applied to. There are also uncertainties with regard to their efficiency, efficacy of tooth movements and cost-effectiveness. Doubts also remain with regard to the predictability of the clinical outcomes and the real-life replication of the software's 3D prediction.

Aside from the fact that patients' compliance is key to successful outcomes, it is well-known that aligners are not very efficient at specific types of tooth movements. The latter include de-rotatory movements, transverse expansion, management of deep bites, root movements and movement of diminutive teeth and teeth with very short clinical crowns [3–5]. These are the same reasons that overcorrections and a combination approach involving both aligners and fixed appliances are frequently recommended. Evidence has only been very recently emerging about the possible use of aligners for more complex cases involving extractions. A trial comparing clear aligners to fixed appliances showed no significant differences in post-treatment Peer Assessment Rating (PAR) scoring nor treatment duration [6].

2.2　Clear Aligners Available

The clinician has now got almost an endless list of brands of aligners to choose from. This chapter intends to describe the most notable of aligner brands; however, it can neither be exhaustive nor be fully comprehensive as brands are continuously innovating their own products launching new aligners and new brands are also being formed in a continuously evolving market. The process commences with the type of aligner selected for use. The classification used, similar to how they have been classified in the section above will be based on the mode of delivery to the patients.

2.2.1　Aligners Manufactured by a Certified Company Involving a Doctor-to-Patient Interface

In alphabetical order, the brands producing these types of aligners include the following:

- 3 M™ Clarity Aligners by 3 M Minnesota, USA
- Accusmile® by Forestadent, Pforzheim, Germany
- Alineadent Aligners by Alineadent, Malaga, Spain
- Angelalign by Angelalign Technology, Inc., Shanghai, China
- CA® Clear Aligners by Scheu-Dental GmbH, Iserlohn, Germany
- ClearCorrect by Straumann Group Basel Switzerland
- eXceed aligners, by eXceed®, Witten, Germany
- EZ-X by DynaFlex®, Missouri, USA

- F22 Aligner by Sweden & Martina, Padua, Italy
- Invisalign by Align Technology, Inc., California, USA
- iROK™ Aligners by iROK™ Digital Dental Studio, California, USA
- K Clear and Clear X by K Line, Düsseldorf-Benrath, Germany
- Nuvola® Clear Aligners by GEO Srl, Vicenza, Italy
- Refine® by TP Orthodontics, Indiana, USA
- Reveal® by Henry Schein, New York, USA
- SLX™Clear Aligner System by Henry Schein, New York, USA
- Smart Moves® by Great Lakes Dental Technologies, New York, USA
- Spark by Ormco™, California, USA
- SureSmile® Dentsply North Carolina, USA
- TwinAligner® Orthocaps System by Rocky Mountains, Indiana, USA

2.2.2 Direct-to-Consumer Aligners Distributed Directly to the Patient

In alphabetical order, the brands producing these types of aligners include the following:

- AlignerCo, New York, USA
- Byte® Aligners, California, USA
- Candid™ Aligners, New York, USA
- NewSmile™ Aligners, Vancouver, British Columbia
- Smile Direct Club™ LLC, Tennessee, USA

2.2.3 In-House Manufacturing by the Treatment Provider

3D printing, over the years has been consistently improving and nowadays has also become available to mainstream businesses including dentistry and orthodontics. The advantages of adopting in-house 3D technology to manufacture aligners is threefold:

  (i) Reduced delivery time
 (ii) Cost-efficiency
(iii) Implementation of a skill-mixed team
(iv) Item customisation
 (v) Design variation

An array of various materials is now available to clinicians who opt to produce aligners in-house. These include stereolithographic materials, epoxy resins, glass-filled polyamides, polylactic acid, acrylonitrile-butadiene-styrene and photopolymers amongst others [7].

2.2.3.1 Pre-printing Process

The initial process invariably starts with a Computer-Aided Design (CAD) model that is obtained after the acquisition of an intraoral scan. This is subsequently modified with the use of a compatible software to the 3D printer which in turn is exported in Standard Tessellation Language (STL) or Object (OBJ) file-readable formats.

Some 3D printers use a laser to cure liquid resin into a hardened form whilst others fuse small particles of polymer powder at high temperatures to build parts. Most users of 3D printers allow them to run unattended until the print is complete. More complex printing machines can also refill the tanks with the necessary material.

2.2.3.2 Post-printing Process

Once the printing of the model has been completed, depending on the type of printer and materials used, several steps would still be needed to attain the final model. The printed parts may require the following:

- Rinsing in alcohol to remove any excess and/or uncured resin from the surfaces
- Further curing to stabilise the mechanical properties
- Manual trimming of the model to eliminate support structures
- Cleaning of the final model

2.2.3.3 Types of Printing Processes

The three most readily accessible types of 3D printers for plastics used for aligner production are as follows:

- Stereolithography (SLA)
- Selective laser sintering (SLS)
- Fused deposition modelling (FDM) also referred to as Fused filament fabrication (FFF)

Both SLA and SLS 3D printers use lasers. In the case of SLA printers, the laser is used to cure liquid resin into hardened plastic in a process called photopolymerisation, whilst in SLS 3D printers the laser is used to sinter small particles of polymer powder into a solid structure.

In the case of FDM/FFF, 3D printers work by extruding thermoplastic filaments through heated nozzles and layering down each level incrementally until the production is completed.

References

1. Jaber ST, Hajeer MY, Burhan AS, Latifeh Y. The effect of treatment with clear aligners versus fixed appliances on Oral health-related quality of life in patients with severe crowding: a one-year follow-up randomized controlled clinical trial. Cureus. 2022;14(5):e25472.
2. Ben Gassem AA. Does clear aligner treatment result in different patient perceptions of treatment process and outcomes compared to conventional/traditional fixed appliance treatment: a literature review. Eur J Dent. 2022;16(2):274–85.

3. Djeu G, Shelton C, Maganzini A. Outcome assessment of Invisalign and traditional orthodontic treatment compared with the American Board of Orthodontics objective grading system. Am J Orthod Dentofacial Orthop. 2005;128(3):292–8. discussion 8.
4. Kravitz ND, Kusnoto B, BeGole E, Obrez A, Agran B. How well does Invisalign work? A prospective clinical study evaluating the efficacy of tooth movement with Invisalign. Am J Orthod Dentofacial Orthop. 2009;135(1):27–35.
5. Li W, Wang S, Zhang Y. The effectiveness of the Invisalign appliance in extraction cases using the ABO model grading system: a multicenter randomized controlled trial. Int J Clin Exp Med. 2015;8(5):8276–82.
6. Jaber ST, Hajeer MY, Burhan AS. The effectiveness of in-house clear aligners and traditional fixed appliances in achieving good occlusion in complex orthodontic cases: a randomized control clinical trial. Cureus. 2022;14(10):e30147.
7. Nguyen TT, Jackson TH. 3D technologies for precision in orthodontics. Semin Orthod. 2018;24:386.

Aligner Treatment Process

3

3.1 Introduction

Any aligner treatment journey partaken by a new patient should be a standardised process, and the pathway should be extremely similar between different patients. The recommended initial step is an initial consultation and evaluation followed by a full dental examination. This is closely followed by acquisition of dental records and the submission of a full prescription by the treating clinician. The patient should be given the opportunity to accept or refuse the proposed treatment via a consenting process. Once the above steps are completed, the clinician will be able to proceed with the submission of the case online, provide treatment, monitor and provide retainers at the end. This chapter will provide an insight into the individual steps involved in an entire treatment journey from start to finish. A greater emphasis is placed on the records part of the journey due to the importance of this phase of treatment.

3.2 The Treatment Journey

The difference between patients' treatment journeys should be negligible or vary minimally if at all. The flow diagram illustrated in Fig. 3.1 demonstrates the entire pathway for a new patient consisting of 11 individual stages.

3.2.1 New Patient Consultation and Evaluation

The first step is a consultation between the treating doctor and the potential new patient. Establishing the complexity of treatment and the possibility of aligner treatment is a fundamental step in initiating the process. Online evaluation tools are available by the aligner manufacturers to support the clinicians' with their decision-making with regard to the grading of complexity of a case.

© The Author(s), under exclusive license to Springer Nature Switzerland AG 2024
S. Abela, *Aligner Systems in Invisible Orthodontics*,
https://doi.org/10.1007/978-3-031-49204-4_3

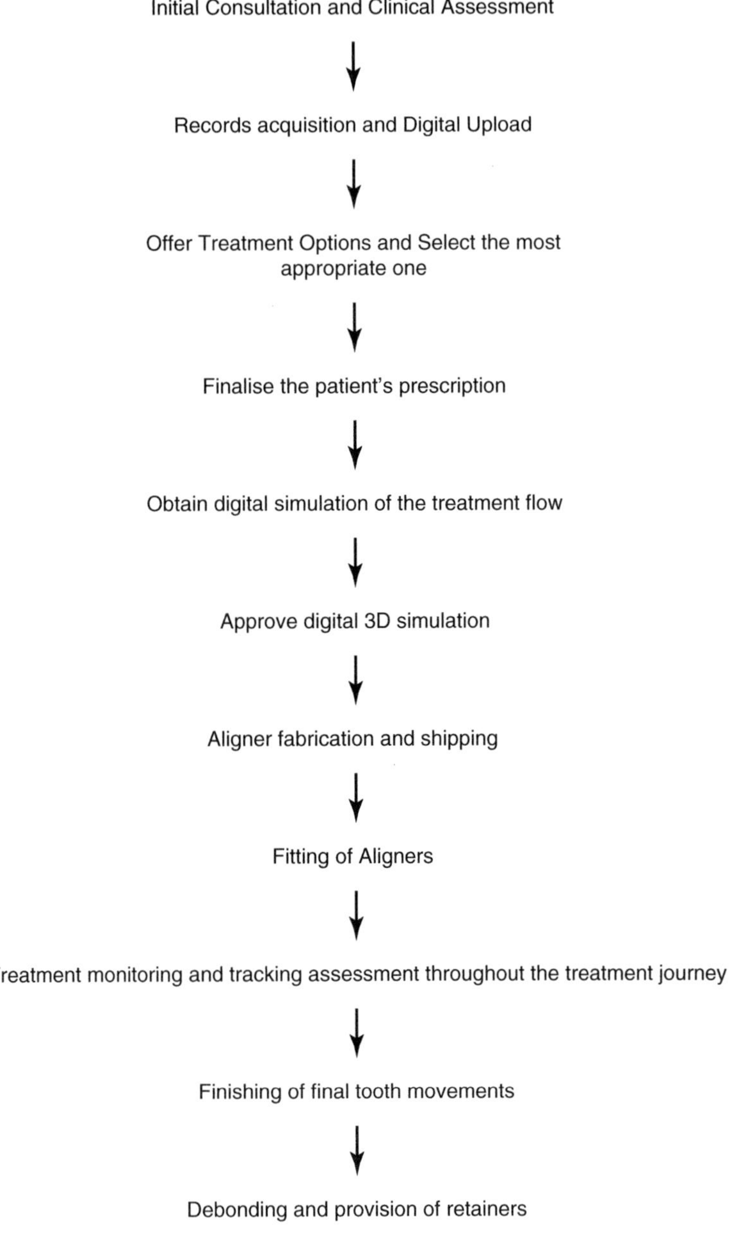

Fig. 3.1 Flow diagram depicting the entire patient journey for aligner treatment

In the case of Align Technology, Inc. (San Jose, Calif., USA) a colour scheme is used to help users differentiate between the different complexities of tooth movement involved; green for simple treatments with very predictable outcomes, blue for moderately difficult cases with variable predictability and black for the least predictable cases with very difficult tooth movements.

3.2.2 Processes Involved for Obtaining and Uploading the Records

The dental records involves obtaining three different aspects of the patient's dentition under examination:

1. Dental impressions for the upper and lower arches
2. Photographic records including extra- and intraoral photographs
3. Dental radiographs

3.2.2.1 Dental Impressions

The purpose for the dental impressions at the beginning of treatment is twofold: study models (SM) and working models (WM) fabrication. Alginate is the impression material classically used for study model production; however, the working models need to be obtained from polyvinyl siloxane (PVS) impression material in heavy body and wash forms. The technique also referred to as putty-wash impression can be obtained as one-stage or two-stage. For most aligner systems, a two-stage approach is preferred. The spacers can be either pre-fabricated or made chair-side allowing at least 2 mm clearance for the wash. The PVS material provides excellent tear strength, maintaining integrity on removal, stability long term and as a result produces a more precise type of impression eliminating remakes. The impressions are then processed by Aligntech's scanners converting them into a digital format with a three-dimensional imagery of the teeth. The format commonly used is Standard Triangle Language (STL) which in turn would need a software package to handle the raw data of the STL format rendering them more user friendly.

Align® provides the clinicians with their own approved impression trays. The sizes available on order are small, medium, large and extra large. The sizes are denoted as S, M, L and XL, respectively, on the tray handle and are all perforated.

3.2.2.2 Digital Dental Scanning

Intraoral scanning is a contemporary way of obtaining arch recording and has modernised impression-taking techniques. It is an alternative to conventional dental impressions with Align Technology, Inc., offering their own brand of intraoral scanners, the iTero scanner range. They currently have the following range of digital scanner products:

- iTero Element Plus Series
- iTero Element Flex
- iTero Element 2
- iTero Element 5D

The scanning process involves the following stages:

- Creating a new patient prescription
- Ensuring a good ergonomic set-up
- Using the correct scanning technique
- Following the recommended scanning protocol
- Utilising the corrective tools available
- Completing the recommended checklist
- Submission of a new case with the appropriate prescription
- Using the 3D viewer to enhance the user's interface

The scanning process is initiated by the user logging into *MyiTero.com* and opening the dashboard allowing the selection of the "New Scan" icon on the screen. A new navigation toolbar appears with four options:

1. To create a new treatment (new patient) or open an existing treatment (existing patient)
2. To enable commencement of scanning
3. To evaluate the scan obtained
4. To send the scan for processing by Align Tech, Inc.

The start of a new treatment entails entering the patient details into the respective fields specifying whether Near InfraRed Imaging (NIRI) is to be used, the type of case being submitted and the lab that the scan should be sent to in case the practitioners is using it for restorative treatment.

In addition, the treatment stage should also be specified. A case is usually considered as a start, mid-treatment or at a final stage where final records are being registered.

The scanning technique should include the entire arch starting from the terminal molar of either side reaching the midline before starting the contralateral side. The scanner head should be rolled from the lingual to the buccal side. Finalisation of the arch should be completed in the anterior region by rolling over the incisors from the lingual to the buccal side similar to the molar region. The "rolling" technique entails the clinician to shift the wand over the occlusal surface from a lingual to a buccal direction maintaining contact with the surface of the tooth at all times to complete the image successfully. In case soft tissue capture is needed, the initial capture should start directly posterior to the central incisors progressing further posteriorly. The intersection between the midline and the dentition should be completed by applying the scanner from the midline to the palatal aspect of the teeth. The soft tissue capture obtainable is clinically useable with evidence available supporting this [1]. On completion of this process for both arches, the clinician should register the scan by obtaining the patient's bite registration. This is captured by asking the patient to replicate the intercuspal position (ICP), and the scanner is placed in the upper and lower premolar region bilaterally and applying a wave-like motion perpendicular to the dentition. In case of multiple bites such as when a functional appliance is needed, this is also possible. The viewing display will annotate the first and second bites as "Both 1" and "Both 2." The clinician has the facility to monitor the time taken to scan and obtain bite registration and also have the deficient areas of the scan highlighted in purple. In case of an oversight where an arch has been missed, a warning message stating "Additional Scans Expected" is also very obvious in the middle of the viewer impeding the clinician from progressing to the next stage. This is very similar in case the bite registration has been overlooked or if a discrepancy between the two sides is detected.

The minimal requirements for acceptance of a scan are as follows:

- An extension of 2 mm gingival tissue scan beyond the zenith of the tooth.
- The entire tooth surface has to be scanned without any deficiencies including the incisor surfaces and occlusal surfaces for the buccal segments.
- The scan should extend to the distal aspect of the terminal tooth (that is the second or third molar).
- An accurate bite registration with the patient in ICP.
- Completion of prescription with all essential details required registered accurately.

Once the capture is completed the clinician has the possibility of correcting and modifying the captured scans before submission. A "fill" option highlights the deficient area by highlighting it and allowing a rescan to "fill" the void. In case of irregularities arising from problems with excessive gingival tissue or gingival exudate, an "Eraser" icon allows this area to be erased to improve the captured image. Another feature is the "Edge Trim" tool which allows for removal of unwanted areas by using a scissors icon. The user also has the facility to delete a section or an arch to be able to rescan it by choosing the "recycle bin" followed by the "broom" icon to control the selected area and once the area is confirmed for deletion, an improved scan will replace the rejected part or arch. Another potential error that can be easily rectified is the bite registration in ICP. Once noticed, by observing the number of contact points within the arch, the user can retake the bite registration.

On submission, the case is available on the Invisalign doctor site after 15 min and is also available on the 3D viewer on the original scanner and on MyiTero.com.

One final option available to the clinician prior to the submission is showing the potential new patient his or her final result by running the Invisalign® Outcome Simulator (IOSim).

3.2.2.3 Dental Photographs

Photographs are also an essential part of record taking. Extra- and intraoral photos are normally taken in order to have a baseline reference to be able to monitor progress during the treatment.

Two options are available for extraoral photographs; Two-dimensional (2D) or three-dimensional (3D). The latter can be used for radiographic superimposition and to establish treatment predictions and soft tissue effects, postoperatively. Intraoral photographs are taken to monitor the tooth movement.

At the start of the treatment, a set of eight photographs is usually the recommended amount; however, nine is also acceptable with the addition of a three-quarter facial view. The reason for taking this photo is that most times, patients are seen by this view rather than at full profile. The set of pre-operative photographs would consist of four extraoral and five intraoral types.

The extraoral photographs needed are:

– Frontal
– Frontal smiling
– Three-quarters view (optional)
– Full profile view

The intraoral photographs needed include:

– Frontal
– Right buccal
– Left buccal
– Upper occlusal view
– Lower occlusal view

Figure 3.2 below is a template showing the ideal mounting of the extra- and intraoral photographs.

Align Technology, Inc. have a downloadable mobile app, Invisalign Photo Uploader which is directly linked to the individual doctor's online platform. This allows clinical usage of the app via the doctor's mobile with automated features and step-by-step instructions on how to use it successfully.

3.2.2.4 Dental X-Rays

X-rays are primarily used for diagnostic purposes. The commonly used X-rays include:

– Periapical radiographs
– Orthopantomogram
– Lateral cephalogram
– Cone beam computed tomography

Periapical radiographs offer excellent diagnostic value. They are very useful in diagnosing dental pathology, bone levels and give an accurate dimension of root lengths. They are not affected by the focal trough and exhibit no distortion in the labial segment region. They can also be taken to determine the precise location of unerupted teeth using the "SLOB" principle' with the describe the parallax technique, an acronym that stands for same lingual and opposite buccal with specific reference to the X-ray tube shift in relation to the ectopic tooth on the image.

Orthopantomograms (OPGs) are advantageous when a general overview of the dentition is needed and for an assessment of the dental development when patients

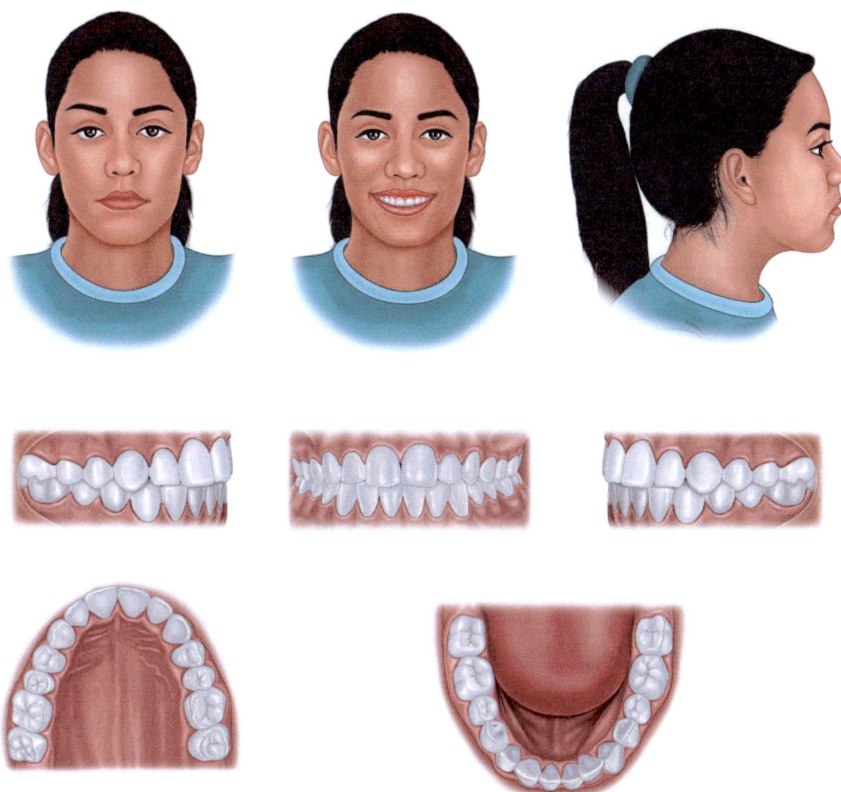

Fig. 3.2 A photographic template showing the ideal mounting of the extra- and intraoral photographs

present in a mixed dentition stage. Although they are not indicated to diagnose decay, carious lesions can also be identified on OPGs. This is indicated in most cases before the start of treatment.

Lateral cephalograms are used to provide an assessment of the skeletal base relation together with the labio-lingual positioning of the incisor teeth to enable precise planning of the tooth movements required. A secondary indication includes the localisation of unerupted teeth.

Cone beam computed tomographs (CBCTs) are fully justified when they are used to augment the diagnostic capability of 2D radiographs. The scope of CBCTs can be fully justified for cases presenting with impacted canines with or without incisor root resorption, impacted teeth close to important oral structures, supernumerary teeth and complete or incomplete alveolar bone clefts.

The specific indication for each type of X-ray can be found in the fourth edition of The Guidelines for the Use of Radiographs in Clinical Orthodontics. The last update was completed in 2015 [2].

3.2.3 Invisalign Product Range

The treating clinician has to be very familiar with the products available for the patient and to be able to choose the product which best suits the patient. The product selected can be for active treatment with an aligner package or passive with Invisalign-designed retainers, Vivera® retainers.

Align Technology, Inc. provide the following the range of aligner products:

1. Express Package consisting of seven consecutive aligners with one additional set of seven aligners to compensate for lack of tracking. The treatment activity duration is 1 year.
2. Lite Package consisting of 14 consecutive aligners with two additional set of 14 aligners included to compensate for lack of tracking. The treatment activity duration is 2 years.
3. Moderate Package consisting of 20 consecutive aligners with two additional sets of up to 20 aligners. The treatment duration is 2 years.
4. Comprehensive Package consisting of as many aligners as needed to reach a clinically acceptable result with additional aligners included in the package until the original targeted result is obtained. The additional aligners have to be ordered prior to the treatment expiration date and the treatment duration is 5 years.
5. Invisalign Teen Package specifically aimed at correcting malocclusions in teenagers with an unlimited amount of trays accounting for mixed dentition phases and transition periods to secondary dentition. Application can start as early as mixed dentition as an interceptive treatment, during a mixed dentition phase and once the secondary dentition is established.
6. Vivera® retainers are the only available retainers by Align Technology, Inc. with claims by the company that they are a third stronger, twice as durable and the patient in the United Kingdom is provided with three sets per jaw to provide long-term retention and have spare retainers at hand in case of loss. They are manufactured using similar 3D imaging and proprietary thermoplastic materials as the aligners.

3.2.3.1 Invisalign Protocol for Placement Hierarchy

The ClinCheck Pro® 6 has a placement prioritisation which is based on the type of individual tooth movement needed. The clinical features presented to the clinician and in turn captured by the software, triggers a cascade of movements based on chronological clinical prioritisation. This allows the software to place the features to obtain movements of the highest importance first followed by those which are less important.

The list of placement in chronological order is as follows:

1. Movement in extraction cases and/or multi-tooth optimised extrusion
2. Root control movement
3. Multi-plane movement such as rotation with or without intrusion or extrusion
4. Extrusion with or without de-rotational movements
5. Optimised support for retention or anchorage for intrusion movements
6. Power ridge feature for Lingual Root Torque (LRT)

The type and amount of tooth movement needed also form the basis for the attachment choice. Attachment placement is denied only in cases where:

- The prescribing doctor eliminates this option
- There are contraindications such as porcelain crowns, gingival hyperplasia, collision with adjacent attachment or small clinical crowns
- ClinCheck® protocol due to associated higher placement hierarchy
- The prescribed tooth movement is minor and does not necessitate the placement of attachments

The latest generation of Invisalign®, G8 with the new SmartForce® Aligner Activation allows the most efficient tooth movement by selecting the surface of the tooth which requires the most surface area of coverage by the aligner for force delivery.

Attachments vary in shape and can be Ellipsoid, Rectangular, Rectangular bevelled and optimised or customised to a specific tooth surface.

The latest software updates allow the treating clinician to vary the attachment configuration in all possible ways. This includes manipulation of the position of each individual attachment, the amount of bevelling and the prominence on the tooth surface.

Figure 3.3 below is an illustration highlighting the type of attachments and the difference in design between ellipsoid and rectangular attachments.

The software allows preferential commands to be pre-set for use with every submission. This allows the clinician to have a pre-set shape and bevelling amount aimed at the individual's preferences for rotational, retention, extrusion and intrusion movements. Attachments instructions can be overridden by the prescribing clinician especially if an increased amount of tray retention is needed. Clinically, this is the norm with diminutive clinical crowns. The attachments serving this purpose can also be placed on the occlusal or lingual surfaces of the teeth.

The ClinCheck Pro® 6 has in-built features to incorporate default attachment shapes. Two such examples include vertical attachments of 1 mm mesial and distal to a central lower incisor for a more efficient space closure protocol. With first premolar extractions, optimised attachments are placed mesial and distal to the extraction site, that is on the canines and second premolars and a conventional attachment of 1 mm thickness on the first molar within the same quadrant.

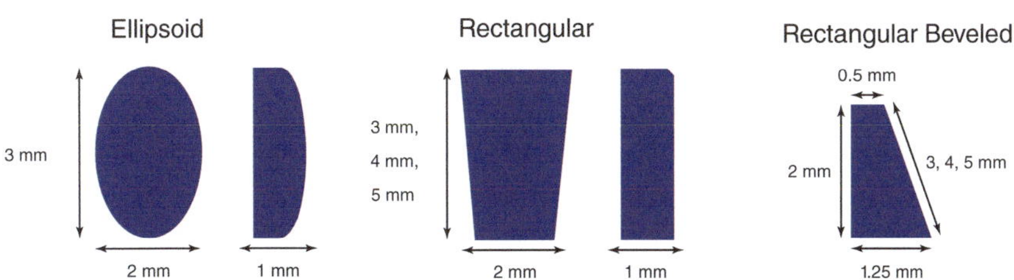

Fig. 3.3 The different types of attachment shapes

3.2.4 Submission of a New Treatment Prescription

Submission of a treatment prescription entails the merging the expectations of a new patient, the doctor's experience together with his or her extensive knowledge of the software and the compliance from both parties.

The process of submission commences on the online platform by selecting the "Start" icon. This is followed by choosing the type of patient based on their age; "Adult," "Teen" or "Child." The choice of the type of patient should be reflected in the clinical findings. For the "Adult" group, the patient should be in an established secondary dentition. In the "Teenage" group, a late mixed or intermediate mixed dentition with unerupted permanent dentition is the norm. The software allows compensation features in the software to predict and enable space analysis. In the "Child" group, a very early mixed dentition is the norm with interceptive treatment being the main reason for treatment prescription. The expectations for this group include eruption of the incisors and first molars at least together with the presence of at least two primary or unerupted teeth in at least three quadrants.

The next step includes choosing between active or passive appliances. For the active appliances and product range, refer to Sect. 3.2.3 above.

The necessary records are taken and uploaded onto the software and the summary of the prescription is confirmed before final submission online. All the necessary materials are packaged in the specific Invisalign shipping box together with disinfected impressions and a copy of the prescription. The shipping label is attached to the outside of the shipping box and a courier service ensures safe delivery to the nearest scanning centre. This process is eliminated if an intraoral scanning technique is used.

Figure 3.4 below illustrates the flow of submission for a new patient.

3.2.5 Creation of 3D ClinCheck® Simulation

The creation of the first 3D simulation of the treatment plan is automated by the software together with the technician. It remains the treating clinicians' responsibility to check the feasibility of obtaining this plan clinically. The ClinCheck® has features to modify the simulation and customise it to the patient's needs based on the biological features, the periodontal and caries status of the patient. The staging tab allows the clinician to visualise the individual tooth movement stages, the attachments and the stage of insertion together with the staging Interproximal Reduction (IPR). The clinicians can also place suggestions for improvement in the comments section of the software with the option of attaching a screenshot of the part of the occlusion being modified.

On submission the software also interprets the level of occlusal contact and allows the clinician to accept them, modify them or allow the software to further correct them. The new 3D simulation will be uploaded onto the online portal for the clinician to recheck and approve.

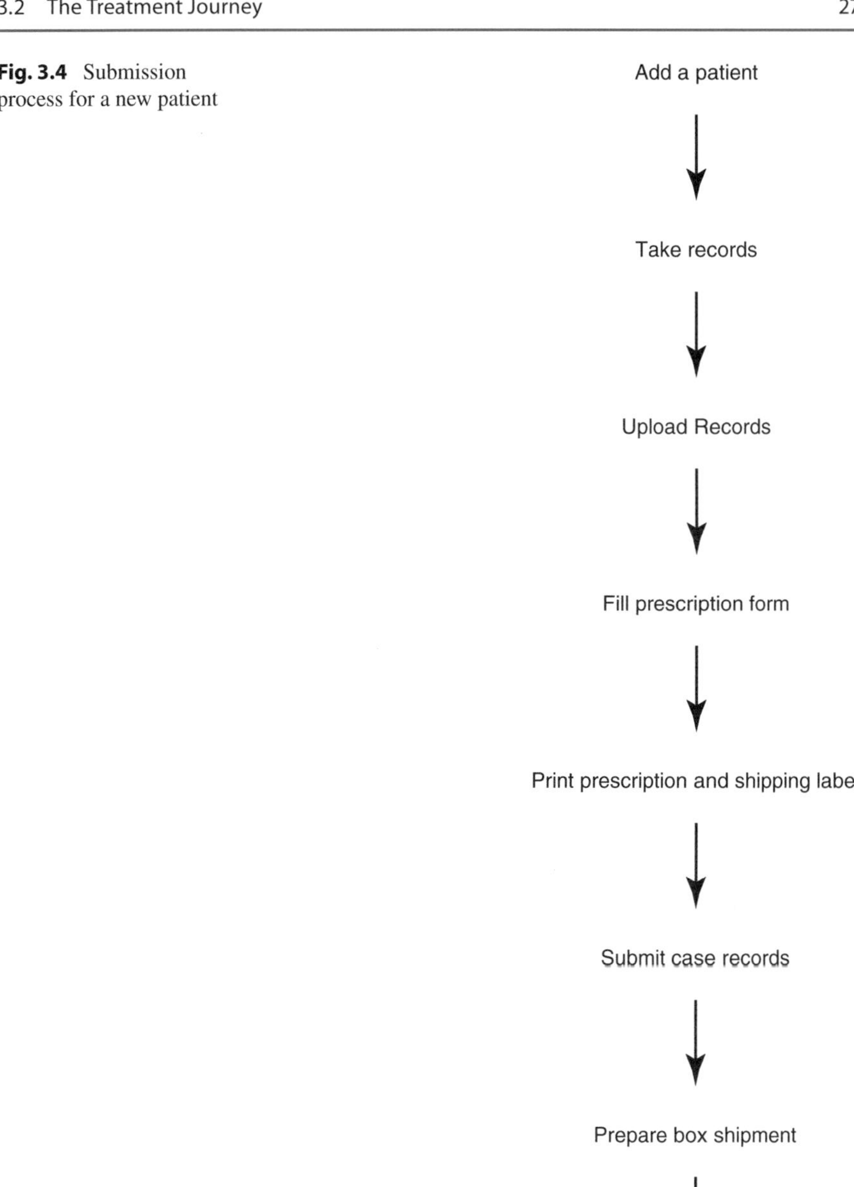

Fig. 3.4 Submission process for a new patient

The tool section of the software has 18 features in total, 5 of which are tabulated data. These are illustrated in Fig. 3.5a, b below.

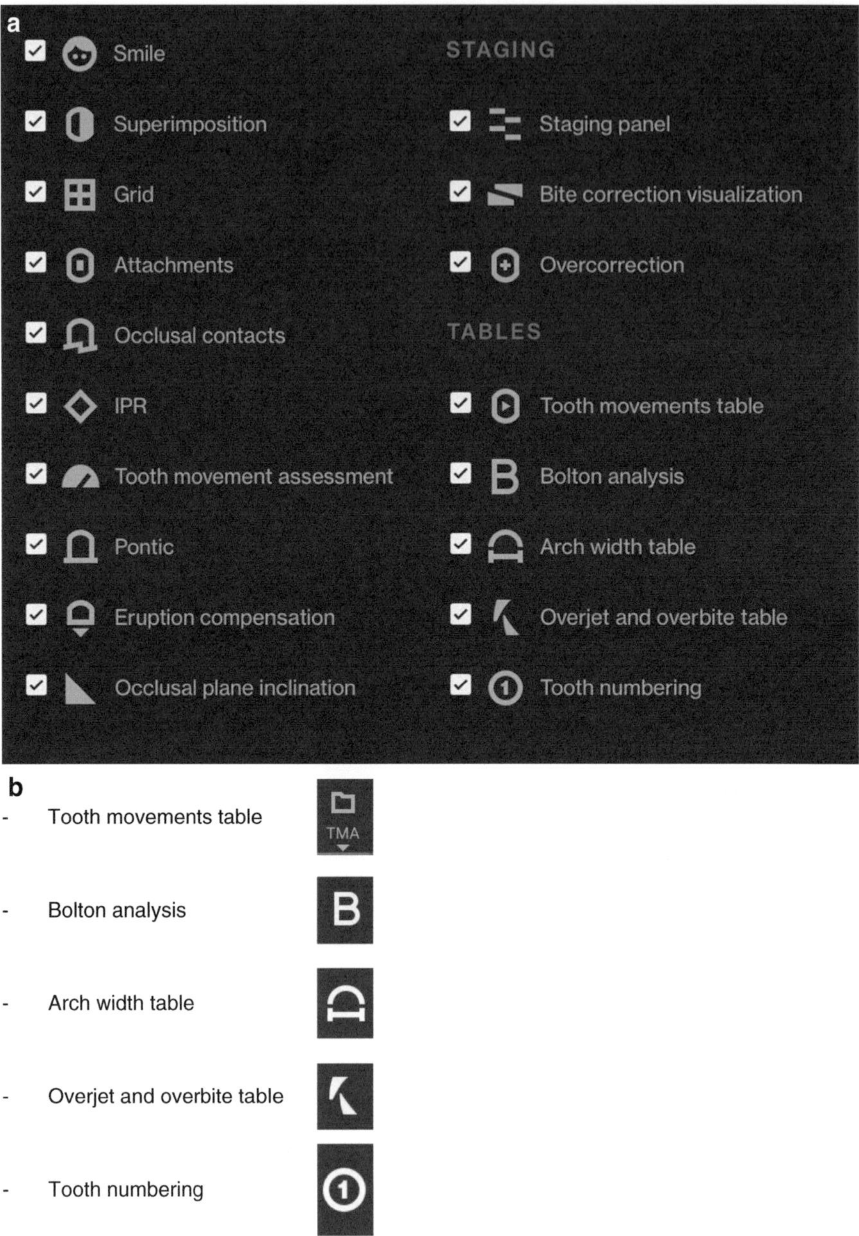

Fig. 3.5 (**a**) The features available on the ClinCheck®. This figure has been reproduced from ClinCheck Pro 6® software and reproduced by kind permission of Align Technology, Inc. (San Jose, Calif., USA). (**b**) The features that appear in tabulated format on the ClinCheck®. This figure has been reproduced from ClinCheck Pro 6® software and reproduced by kind permission of Align Technology, Inc. (Santa Clara, Calif., USA)

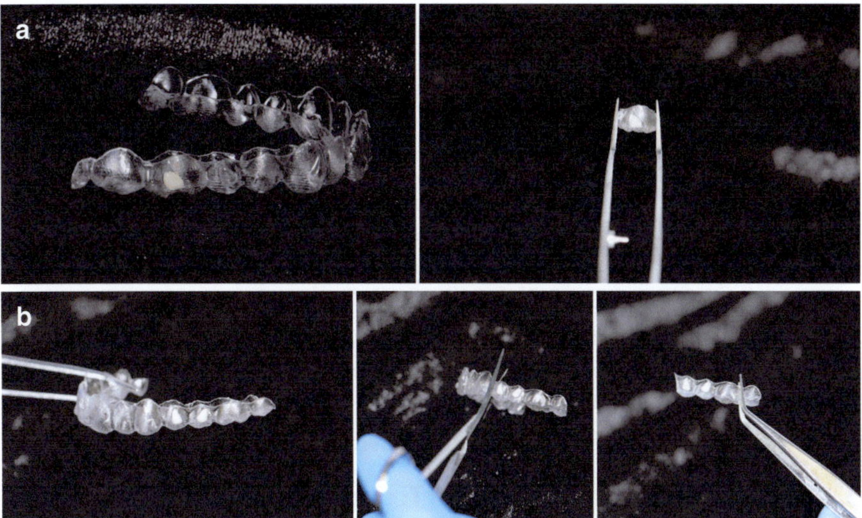

Fig. 3.6 (**a**) Illustrates the sectional trimming of a molar tooth from the original template to replacing a lost attachment on this tooth. (**b**) Illustrates the sectional trimming of the original template to replace two premolar attachments. This figure has been reproduced by kind permission of the author, Dr. Stefan Abela

The features that can be made available to the clinician are shown below. Ticking the box will allow the feature to be visualised during the treatment plan simulation forecast.

Additional features included in a tabulated format are listed below in Fig. 3.6b. Each of the above tabulated data are preceded by a sign pertaining to the individual movements. The signs are shown next to each value above.

3.2.6   ClinCheck® Approval by the Clinician

The clinicians' role in formulating a treatment plan using the iCloud-based software is key to the treatment's success. The step-by-step process is discussed in detail in Chap. 5 below.

3.2.7   Tray Fabrication and Shipping

The manufacturing process is an automated system. Pressing the "approval" icon on the software initiates this process with digital instruction being directly relayed to the manufacturing plant.

Shipping is done via the authorised courier and will be shipped to the clinicians' practice as registered on the portal.

3.2.8　Starting the Treatment

At the fitting stage, the clinician ensures good fit. The latter is defined by a flush fit of the aligner with the teeth. Any "voids," spacing between the tray and the teeth will result in a deficit in the pre-programmed tooth movement, technically referred to as "tracking." The main causes for lack of tracking is as follows:

- Decreased amount of wear or decreased compliance by the wearer
- Lack of IPR or other instructions included in the plan
- Damage to the aligners
- Inappropriate insertion resulting in voids between the aligners and tooth surface
- Loss of attachments or loss of attachment material that decreases the contact surface area between the teeth and the linter

3.2.9　Monitoring the Progress of Treatment

The treatment progress can be monitored face to face or by virtual means. Both types should encourage the clinician to follow a routine to ensure progress is on par with the pre-determined sequence as visualised on the software.

The monitoring process should include the following stages:

- Assessment of the aligner fit
- Cross-checking of the clinical findings with the 3D ClinCheck® simulation
- Assessment of attachment shape and volume
- Assessment of amount of IPR carried out and related to the prescribed amount on the ClinCheck®
- The need to relieve areas of the trays, buccally or lingually, which are causing mucosal trauma
- The presence of buttons or precision cuts for the placement of elastic bands as prescribed on the ClinCheck®
- The need to place new attachments as more tooth movement is obtained

3.2.9.1　Clinical Management of Lost Attachments

Loss of attachments is normal and acceptable during a course of treatment. Early loss of all of the attachments is reflective of a bonding failure and the process should be repeated; however, singular attachments can be replaced by trimming off the original template provided to accommodate the tooth onto which a new attachment is needed.

A replacement template can be ordered directly from the manufacturer. Standard debridement, isolation, bonding and placement of composite resin should be loaded into the template and light-cured for 20 s.

In more advanced stages of treatment, the original template will be ill-fitting and the template should be trimmed in the individual tooth sections and applied very similarly to the pre-formed plastic crowns used in restorative dentistry. Figure 3.6 below illustrates this technique.

3.2.9.2 Clinical Management of Tracking Issues

Lack of "tracking" due to non-ideal fitting of the trays on the teeth gives rise to undesired tray to tooth-surface contact which displaces a tooth or teeth in a different position from the predicted one on the software.

A tracking problem defined as the amount of discrepancy between the tooth surface and the tray can be classified as mild, moderate or severe. The clinical management will in turn depend on the magnitude of the tracking problem.

Mild tracking problem: A very minimal discrepancy considered to be less than 1 mm.

Clinical Solution/s:

(a) Ensure compliance
(b) Increase aligner wear time to 22 h a day
(c) Increase the interval between tray changes
(d) Introduce aligner seaters also known chewies

Moderate Tracking Problem: A minimal degree of discrepancy between 1 and 2 mm.

Clinical Solution/s:

(a) Apply solutions mentioned above for mild tracking problems.
(b) Use detailing pliers.
(c) Introduce auxiliaries such as buttons to approximate a tooth closer to the aligner, to facilitate de-rotations or to alter a root tip by placing the button as close to the cervical aspect of the tooth as possible.

Severe Tracking Problem: A significant degree of discrepancy greater than 2 mm.

Clinical Solution/s:

(a) Apply solutions mentioned above for mild and moderated tracking problems
(b) Take new dental impressions or intraoral scans to order a refinement batch

iTero™ allows the possibility to trace the origin of the tracking problem using "Time Lapse" giving the clinician the opportunity to modify the cause of the problem. The aligners are covered with a warranty which can be activated in cases where the fit is not satisfactory.

The only exception to accepting a gap between the aligner and the incisor aspect of a tooth is the upper lateral incisors fitted with optimised root control attachments.

3.2.10 Finalisation of Treatment

The monitoring cycle gets completed at this stage of treatment followed by the removal of the attachments, polishing and provision of retainers.

3.2.11 The Retention Phase

Although to some, this phase is not considered as part of the treatment, the retention phase should be considered as a continuation of the active treatment.

Retention is the provision of retainers which aim at preventing unwanted tooth movement following active orthodontic treatment.

The retainers manufactured by Align Technology, Inc. are called Vivera retainers and are also made of a different thermoplastic material to the active trays, designed solely to be used after the active phase of orthodontic treatment. The use of retainers following orthodontic treatment is a recommendation that should not be avoided as a degree of unwanted movement is always expected.

Align Technology, Inc. relays the following advantages of Vivera retainers over similar type of retainers by other manufacturers:

- Decreased retainer wear as three sets are supplied
- Stronger than similar retainers from other manufacturers by up to 30%
- Ability to correct minor relapses due to the strength conferred by the proprietary material
- Can be ordered with or without lingual fixed retainers
- Can be ordered with pontics to camouflage missing teeth
- Enables good levels of oral hygiene
- Can be prescribed to non-invisalign patients

References

1. Deferm JT, Schreurs R, Baan F, Bruggink R, Merkx MAW, Xi T, et al. Validation of 3D documentation of palatal soft tissue shape, color, and irregularity with intraoral scanning. Clin Oral Investig. 2018;22(3):1303–9.
2. Isaacson K, Thom AR. Orthodontic radiography guidelines. Am J Orthod Dentofacial Orthop. 2015;147(3):295–6.

Biomechanics with Aligner Treatment

4

4.1   Introduction

The introduction of SmartForce® in 2020 led to more innovations in the biomechanical aspect of clear aligner therapy. This innovation is based on the information database collected by Align Technology, Inc. (San Jose, Calif, USA) based on previously treated patients. In its current iteration, generation number eight, referred to as G8, Invisalign in conjunction with SmartForce® allowed the company to claim that this combination produces the optimal force delivery to teeth by directing the amount and directing the forces where needed leading to minimal unwanted tooth movement.

4.2   SmartForce®

SmartForce®, claimed by the manufacturers as the ultimate in aligner material, was produced to offer advantageous benefits over its predecessor including better tooth movement efficiency.

4.2.1   Definition

By definition, the force delivery with SmartForce® allows total customisation and tailor-made forces to the needs of the patient being treated. Tooth movement is delivered through precisely delivered forces which are tailored to the individual needs. The design and direction of these forces are software-led which in turn are based on the clinical presentations and clinical preferences of the treating clinicians.

The design features that make up SmartForce® are discussed in the section below.

© The Author(s), under exclusive license to Springer Nature Switzerland AG 2024
S. Abela, *Aligner Systems in Invisible Orthodontics*,
https://doi.org/10.1007/978-3-031-49204-4_4

4.2.2 Features

The optimised features and attachments included in G8 with SmartForce® does not necessarily allow the aligner material to conform to the surface of the attachment. The shape of the aligner is determined by the software to allow the right amount and direction of force activation. Any gaps are intentionally placed in non-active surfaces to allow clearance for more effective tooth movement.

4.2.2.1 Buccal Power Ridges (BPRs)

BPRs® as the name suggests is a feature within the gingival third of the buccal aspect of the aligner. It is used on upper and lower incisors and produces lingual root torque, LRT. The threshold for use is that of 3 ° of LRT with 1 ° of LRT per aligner. BPRs can be coupled with lingual power ridges. This feature is placed on upper incisors due to the larger anatomical crown and produces lingual root torque and incisor retraction at 1 ° and 0.25 mm, respectively. Figure 4.1 illustrates BPRs.

4.2.2.2 Optimised Rotation Attachments

In contrast to conventional attachments, optimised attachments allow a tailored movement based on the patient's specific needs.

This is used on upper and lower canines and premolars. It is designed to facilitate de-rotation with an introduction threshold of 5 ° with 2 ° of correction per aligner. Figure 4.2 illustrates this type of attachment.

Fig. 4.1 Illustrates the placement of BPR on the buccal and lingual aspect of an incisors with the inset showing how it is seen on the tray

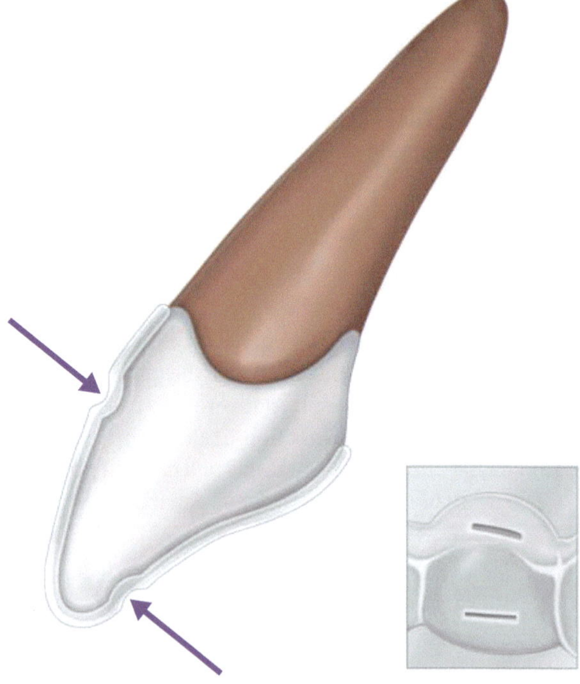

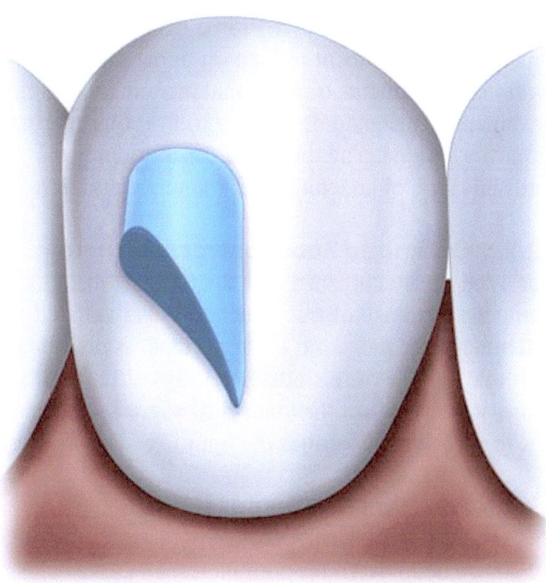

Fig. 4.2 Illustrates an optimised rotation attachment

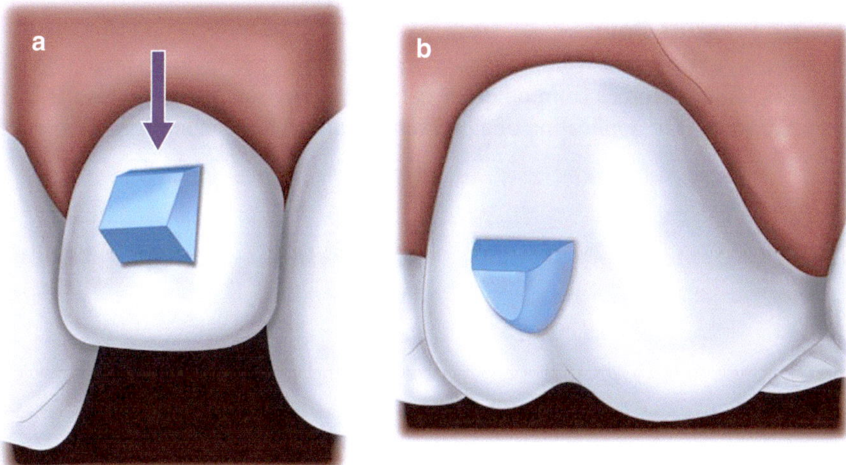

Fig. 4.3 (**a** and **b**) Illustrate an optimised extrusion attachment for anterior or posterior teeth

4.2.2.3 Optimised Extrusion Attachments

This type of attachment is optimised to produce extrusion movements. It is indicated for upper and lower incisors and canines; however, it can also be used for premolars and molars, albeit in a different shape to conform with the requirements of the anatomical variation. The software's threshold for this attachment introduction is 0.5 mm with 0.2 mm of movement achieved per aligner. The same is applicable for multi-tooth extrusion with the attachments being placed on multiple incisors. Figure 4.3 below illustrates optimised extrusion attachments.

4.2.2.4 Optimised Multi-Plane Attachment

This type of attachment is used on upper lateral incisors for extrusion, tipping and rotational movements or rotational movements together with intrusion or excursion movements. Designed differently to fit molar morphology, it can be used on upper and lower molars. The threshold for introduction is 5 °. Figure 4.4a, b below illustrates this type of attachments for anterior and posterior teeth.

4.2.2.5 Optimised Root Control Attachment

This type of attachment is used on upper incisors, upper and lower canines and premolars. The use of this attachment is indicated to provide dual and synergistic attachments on the same tooth surface to provide mesio-distal root tipping. The threshold for use of this attachment is 0.75 mm of mesio-distal tipping around the centre of resistance of the tooth and progress can be expected at 0.25 mm per aligner. Figure 4.5 below illustrates the optimised root control attachment.

4.2.2.6 Precision Bite Ramps (PBRs)

Placed on the palatal aspect of the upper incisors, precision bite ramps are designed to manage deep overbites with increased curves of Spee.

Refer to Sect. 8.4.2 for further details about PBRs. Figure 4.6 below illustrates the use of PBRs.

4.2.2.7 Pressure Points

Pressure areas designed within the aligner to act on a specific tooth area, together with the resultant forces from other areas of the aligner on the tooth, results in an intrusive force. The application of a pressure point can be seen in Fig. 4.7 below.

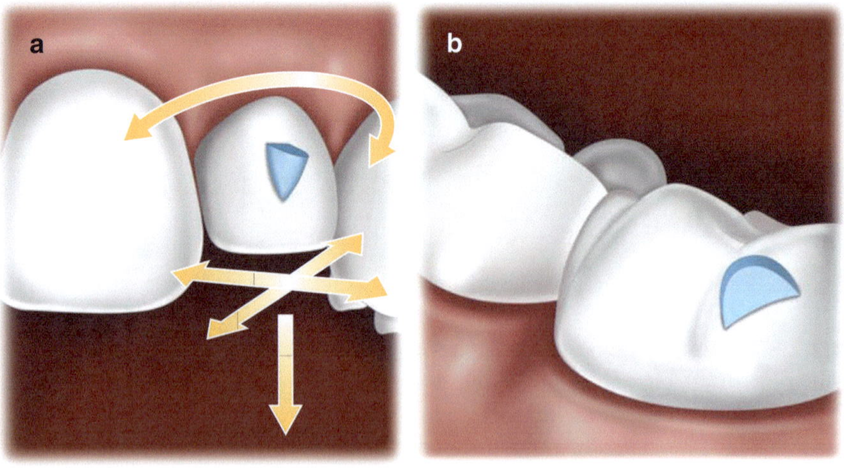

Fig. 4.4 Illustrates an optimised multi-plane attachment for anterior teeth (**a**) and posterior teeth (**b**)

Fig. 4.5 Illustrates an optimised root control attachment for anterior teeth

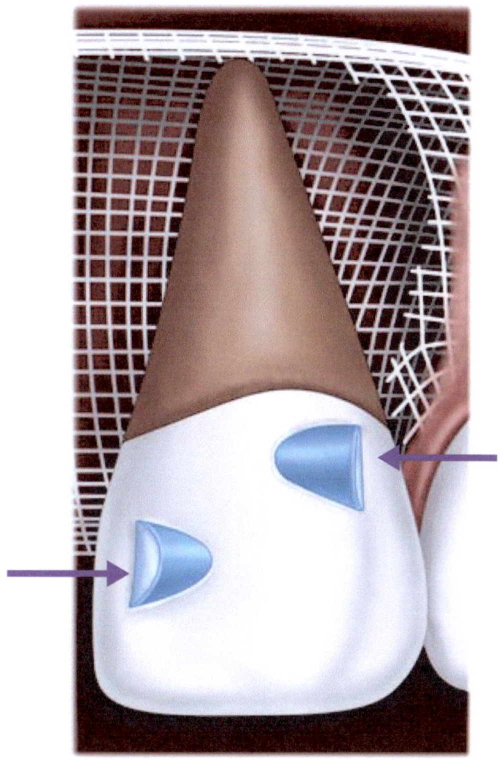

Fig. 4.6 Illustrates precision bite ramps placed on the palatal aspect of the teeth in the upper labial segment

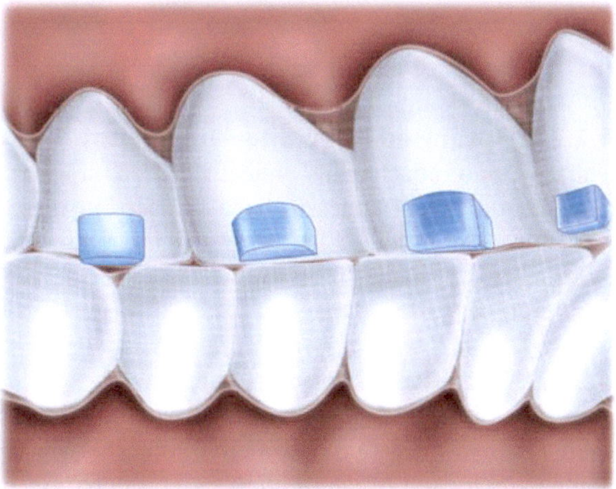

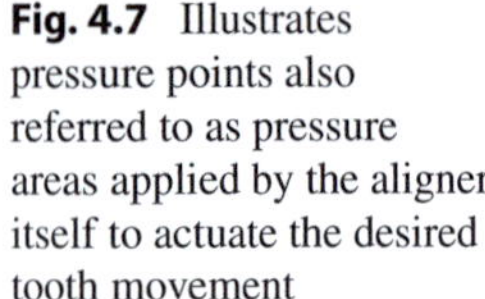

Fig. 4.7 Illustrates pressure points also referred to as pressure areas applied by the aligner itself to actuate the desired tooth movement

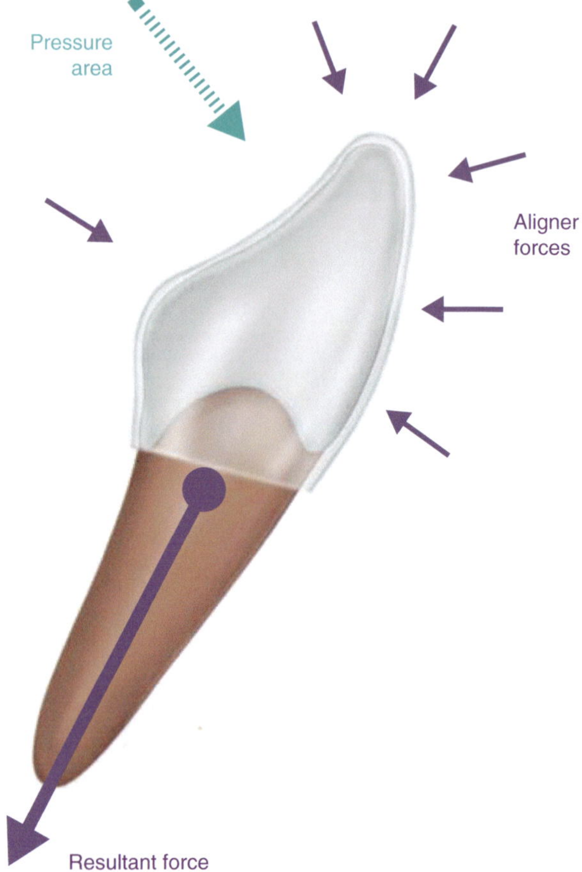

4.2.2.8 Optimised Deep Bite Attachment

These types of attachments typically placed on lower premolars although can also be placed on lower canines are used for deep bite management cases. A complementary movement to lower incisor intrusion is premolar extrusion which this type of attachment is primarily used for. An optimised deep bite attachment can be visualised in Fig. 4.8.

4.2.2.9 Optimised Support Attachment

This type of attachment is indicated when reciprocal anchorage or movement is used. Such an indication is evident during intrusion of central incisors when concomitant extrusion of lateral incisors is needed. An optimised support attachment can be seen in Fig. 4.9.

4.2.2.10   Multi-Tooth Unit Optimised Retraction Attachment

Used on upper and lower canines for canine retraction, this type of attachment is indicated in first premolar extraction planned to provide additional anchorage or for posterior mesial movement. The use of a multitooth unit optimised retraction attachment can be seen in Fig. 4.10.

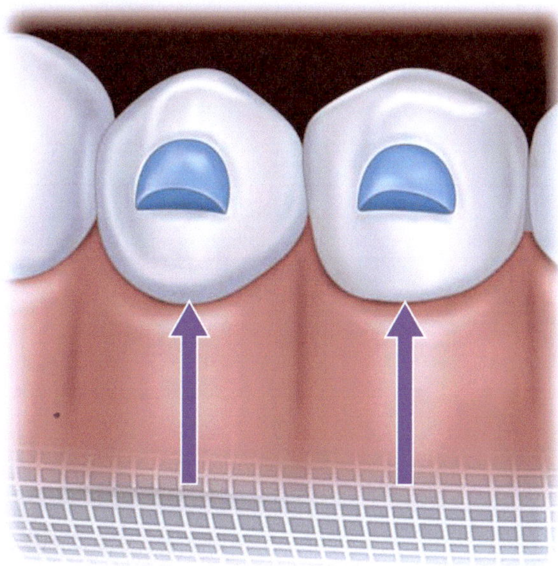

Fig. 4.8 Illustrates optimised deep bite attachments on lower premolars to flatten the curve of Spee, an important aspect of deep bite management

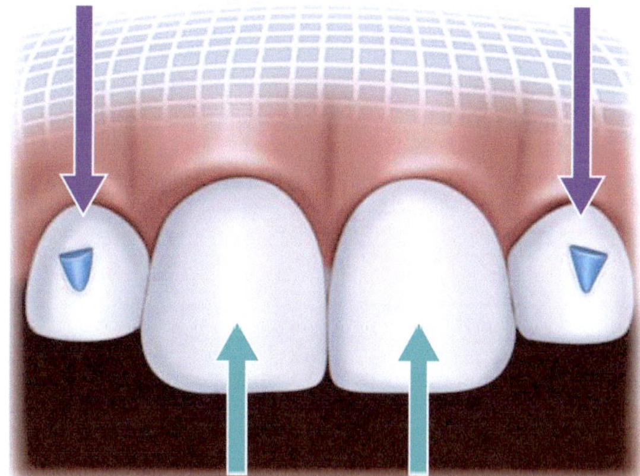

Fig. 4.9 Illustrates optimised support attachments on upper lateral incisors to obtain reciprocal anchorage in cases that present with vertical discrepancies anteriorly

4.2.2.11 Multi-Tooth Unit Optimised Maximum or Moderate Anchorage Attachment

Used on upper and lower second premolars and molars, they are indicated for first premolar extraction cases to provide additional anchorage or up to 2 mm posterior mesial movement. A multi-tooth unit optimised maximum anchorage attachment can be seen in Fig. 4.11 below.

4.2.2.12 Optimised Anchorage Attachment

These attachments are used in upper molars and second premolars. They aid incisor retraction with a threshold movement of 1 mm with 0.2 mm of movement per aligner. Figure 4.12 below illustrates the optimised anchorage attachment.

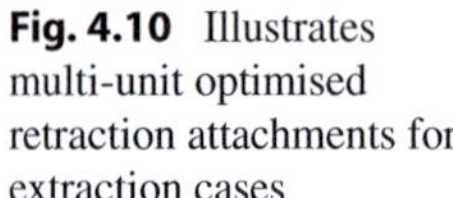

Fig. 4.10 Illustrates multi-unit optimised retraction attachments for extraction cases

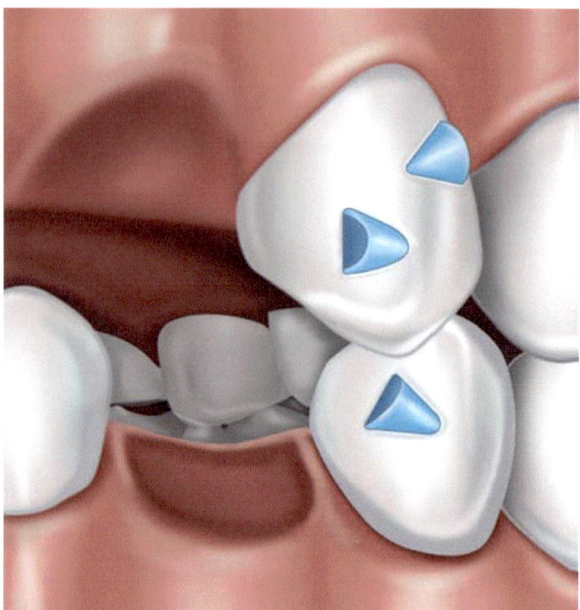

Fig. 4.11 Illustrates multi-unit optimised moderate anchorage attachments on molars

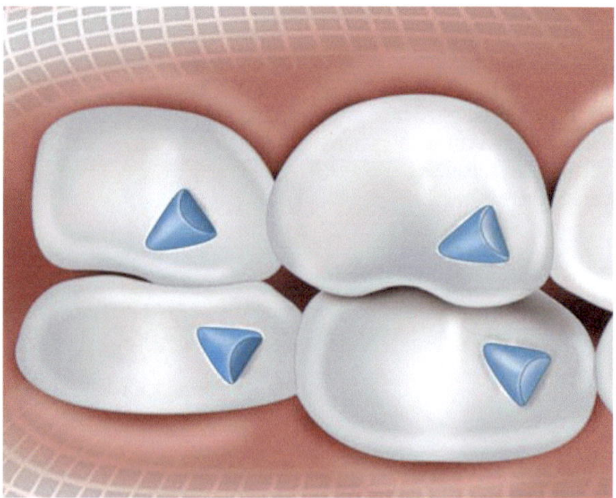

4.2.2.13   Optimised Expansion Support Attachment

New to generation eight, this feature is available on upper and lower premolars and first molars. It facilitates expansion and could be combined with rotational movements. The software's threshold for introduction of this feature is 0.5 mm of crown expansion and 5 ° of rotation. Individual aligners obtain this movement with a paced progress of 0.25 mm and 2 ° with each change.

In contrast to previous generations, Invisalign® G8 produces less tipping with these types of attachments. This is due to the resultant synergistic combination of forces between the optimised attachment and the aligner. The counterforces generated across the centre of resistance of molars, located at the furcation area, produces

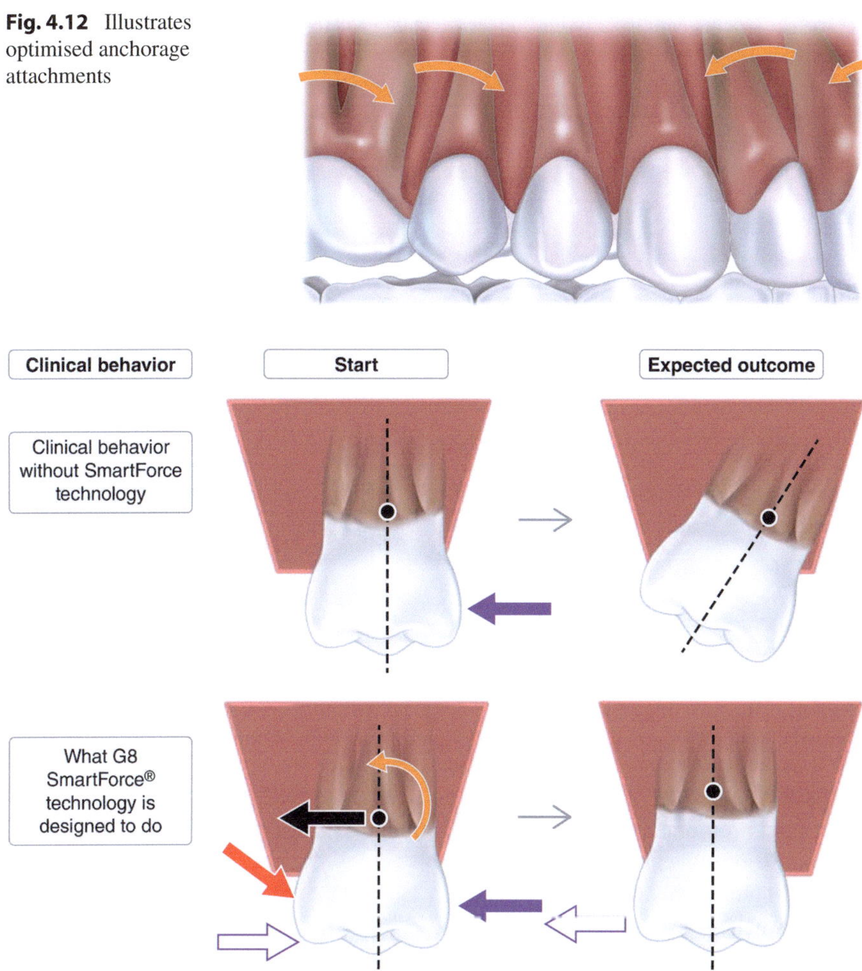

Fig. 4.12 Illustrates optimised anchorage attachments

Fig. 4.13 Illustrates optimised anchorage attachments providing support during expansion movements to prevent excessive buccal tipping of the molars with concomitant interferences resulting from palatal cusps prematurely contacting the occlusal surfaces of the lower counterparts

less tipping effects. Figure 4.13 below illustrates optimised support attachments during expansion movements.

4.2.3 Prioritisation of Attachment Placement

In cases needing multiple attachments, the software will automatically prioritise the attachments that need to be placed first. In some instances, different attachments will not be able to be placed on the same aligner and will be introduced in different stages of treatment.

The prioritisation by the software in listed in numerical order below:

Table 4.1 Tabulation of the attachment placement protocol as per Align Technology, Inc. (Santa Clara, Calif., USA) ClinCheck Pro 6® protocol

Tooth movement	Rotation	Extrusion	Intrusion	Mesio/distal root tip	Retention	Lingual root torque (LRT)
Upper central incisors	N/A	OEA	LPA	ORCA	N/A	For LRT only: BPRF For LRT and retraction: Dual BPRF and LPRF
Upper lateral incisors	OMPA	OEA (single or multi-tooth)	LPA	ORCA	Optimised support	For LRT only: BPRF For LRT and retraction: Dual BPRF and LPRF
Lower incisors	N/A	OEA	LPA	N/A	N/A	BPRF
Upper and lower canines	ORA	OEA	LPA	ORCA	ODBA	N/A
Upper and lower premolars	ORA	OEA	N/A	ORCA	ODBA	N/A
Upper and lower molars	OMPA	OEA	N/A	N/A	ODBA	N/A

Abbreviations: *N/A* not applicable, *BPRF* buccal power ridge feature, *LPA* lingual pressure area, *LPRF* lingual power ridge feature, *ODBA* optimised deep bite attachment, *OEA* optimised extrusion attachment, *OMPA* optimised multi-plane attachment, *ORA* optimised rotational attachment, *ORCA* optimised root control attachment

First: First premolar extraction and multi-tooth extrusion movements.
Second: Root movements (mesial-distal).
Third: Single tooth vertical and rotation.
Fourth: Anchorage for intrusion.
Fifth: Power ridge feature for LRT.

4.2.4   Summary of SmartForce® Attachment Placement Protocol

The summary of the SmartForce® attachment protocol during placement has been tabulated in Table 4.1 below.

4.3   Customising the Biomechanics

The flat surface of an attachment is the active surface to which an aligner binds to and produces the necessary moment of force.

The biomechanics might not necessarily be the same throughout the treatment and any variation in force will get actuated through a difference in the interaction between the aligner and the attachment. The more the aligner interacts at an angle to the attachment the greater the force and vice versa. This allows control of the force magnitude.

For changes in root angulation, two forces are generally needed to control tipping forces and allow changes in root angulation. In this case, the attachments placed need to produce two forces: one greater than the other. The larger force is created by a greater difference in interaction or mismatch between the aligner and the attachment as discussed above. This force must be in the direction of the tooth movement wanted. The generation of the smaller force with the second set of attachments is further away from the centre of resistance creating a larger moment of force which in turn allows controlled root angulation changes. If the two forces created are equal in magnitude, the resultant moment of force would be a force couple, usually beneficial in de-rotating teeth.

In addition to SmartForce®, SmartTrack™ and SmartStage technologies provide a more predictable biomechanical strategy to the clinician.

In general terms, the three favoured materials for aligner manufacture is thermoplastic polyurethane (TPU), polypropylene (PP), and polyester (PE) [1]. Polyethylene terephthalate glycol (PET-G), polyethylene terephthalate (PET), and polycarbonate (PC) are also in use; however, TPU remains the most versatile material to date, and hence its use by Align Technology, Inc. and the introduction of SmartTrack™ material. The thickness can range from 0.5 mm to 1.5 mm. The thickness is directly relevant to their stress relaxation properties.

Any other aligner material under consideration by any manufacturer should be introduced in context of the ideal aligner properties for optimal force delivery. These include the following:

1. Delivery of gentle constant force
2. Correct stiffness
3. Ideal stress relaxation
4. Transparent
5. Smooth
6. Inexpensive
7. Long shelf-life
8. Non-toxic and safe for oral use
9. Dimensionally stable with no degradation and no deformation
10. Biodegradable over time or recyclable to allows safe disposal

The stress relaxation properties of an aligner originates from the material used to construct the tray from. In case of Invisalign® aligners, the product name used is EX30, short for Exceed. For Vivera® retainers and Invisalign® templates the product names are EX40 and EX15, respectively. Exceed has superseded Proceed 30 (PC30) in 2013 due to shortcomings in its physical properties and failing to meet the requirements needed for successful force delivery intraorally.

The composition of the material is polyurethane from methylene diphenyl diisocyanate and 1,6 hexanediol. This material fully is tested under the United States of Pharmacopeia regulations and has its safety data sheet available online via the following url; https://c3-preview.prosites.com/242082/wy/docs/MSDS_Aligner_ Material_EX30_Vivera_Templates.pdf.

The document is entitled: "MSDS (Material Safety Data Sheet) for Invisalign Appliance Materials - EX15, EX30 and EX40", document number 2088." The last print is dated; 1st of July 2013.

The change from PC30 to EX30 changed the characteristics of the aligners with different stress-strain characteristics, with the latter capable of providing more suitable force delivery for the purposes intended. The elasticity reported was one and a half times greater.

EX30 was eventually replaced with the SmartTrack™ material; LD30 had claimed improvements in flexibility, fracture resistance and transparency. The main component added to EX30 was an elastomer for an enhanced oral performance however with acquired disadvantages mainly that of increased hydrophilic properties especially in the presence of lowered PHs and increased bacterial conglomeration [2]. Further scientific data highlights the potential mechanical, chemical and morphological changes during intraoral use rendering the predicted to actual outcome ratio less predictable [3].

SmartTrack™ is still based on methylene diphenyl diisocyanate and 1,6 hexanediol however has been modified with the addition of additives to modify the characteristics as described above. The LD30 thickness for Invisalign® trays is 0.75 mm whilst the EX40 and EX15 thickness for Vivera® and Invisalign® templates, respectively, remains the same at 1.02 mm and less than 0.75 mm.

A randomised controlled trial by Bruno et al. in 2021 identified the superiority of Spark™ template over Invisalign® template in transferring attachments to the surfaces of teeth, resulting in fewer attachments debonding [4].

Different chemical structures are used by different aligner manufacturers. The list below although not exhaustive, outlines some of the more common polymer used ones:

1. Zendura™—Thermoplastic Polyurethane manufactured by Bay Materials LLC, Fremont, California, United States
2. Clear Correct®—Polyurethane manufactured by Straumann group AG, Basel, Switzerland
3. Biolon®—PET-G (Polyethylene terephthalate glycol) manufactured by Dreve Dentamid GmbH. Unna, Germany
4. Duran®—PET (Polyethylene terephthalate) manufactured by Scheu dental, Iserlohn, Germany
5. easyDU©—PET (PFb/PFc) manufactured by BenQ AB DentCare Corporation, Taipei, Taiwan
6. F22—Polyurethane manufactured by Sweden and Martina SpA, Due Carrare, Padua, Italy
7. Invisalign® SmartTrack™—Multi-layer aromatic thermoplastic polyurethane manufactured by Align Technology, Inc., Santa Clara, California, United States
8. MaxFlex™—TPU manufactured by Maxflex Medical Technology Co., Shanghai, China

9. Nuvola®—PET-G (Polyethylene terephthalate glycol) manufactured by GEO srl, Rome, Italy
10. Spark™—Trugen (multi-layer polyurethane) manufactured by Ormco™Corporation, Orange, California, United States

The mechanical properties of an aligner material have to include enough hardness to prevent intraoral deterioration; however, it has to also demonstrate enough elasticity to provide a gentle continuous force as described above.

These properties are not only dependent on the molecular structure of the various materials but also on the changes they undergo during the thermoforming process.

The modulus of elasticity for Invisalign® aligners have been measured at between 2200 and 2500 MPa. This is in line with the expected values of 2000–2500 MPa albeit slightly higher. Higher elasticity properties could lead to more intraoral deformation from the repetitive occlusal loading.

4.4   Factors Affecting the Biomechanics

The four predominant aligner factors that translate and actuate the physical tooth movements from the 3D simulation to real live are as follows:

1. The use or not of attachments [5]
2. The type of thermoplastic material used [6]
3. The thickness of the aligner material [7]
4. The physical properties of the material and its associated degenerative changes in the intraoral environment [8]
5. The manufacturing method of the aligner material [9]

In two separate studies comparing six different aligners, findings highlighted the commonalities between the different types. These include all the types of aligners tested showed a good overall fit although the material thickness tended to be greatest in the posterior regions in comparison to anterior regions. The aligners showed tendencies to be thicker occlusal than gingival and the fitting of the aligners over the anterior teeth was more accurate in comparison to the more posterior teeth. F22 by Sweden Martin, Padua, Italy was the most consistent of the six types of aligners included in these two studies [7, 10]. Being knowledgeable of the above phenomena offers the clinician an explanation into the differences in the degree of tooth movement experienced in vivo and the differences in the stages of onset of tooth movement between different segments.

4.5   Finishing and Detailing with Aligner Treatment

Finishing is a key stage of treatment and below are a few finishing techniques that can be very useful to the clinician when this stage of treatment is reached.

4.5.1   Overcorrectors

The clinician has the possibility to prescribe overcorrectors at the end of treatment to ensure additional orthodontic tooth movement specifically to areas which have been anticipated as difficult to correct. Overcorrectors, usually 1–3 in number are active trays producing additional tooth movement. This term could be confused with the actual overcorrection in the prescription to overcome a decreased amount of real-life movement when compared to the simulation on the software.

A clinical tip is that overcorrectors are prescribed for teeth that are known to exhibit greater discrepancies between virtual and real life. This includes canines and premolars in contrast to incisors which have a flatter crown morphology. It is also advisable to review the patient prior to dispensing these trays to confirm the need as they might lead to excessive tooth movement which is also undesirable.

4.5.2   Overcorrection

The term overcorrection refers to the amount of excessive tooth movement that should be incorporated in the software to compensate for the inconsistencies between the 3D projections on the software to real life. Several studies have shown this repeatedly with a mean accuracy averaging around 50% [11–13]. The mean efficacy of tooth movement with aligners is illustrated in Fig. 4.14 below. Being knowledgeable of the tooth movements that are not replicated successfully the clinicians can prescribe overcorrection to overcome this shortcoming.

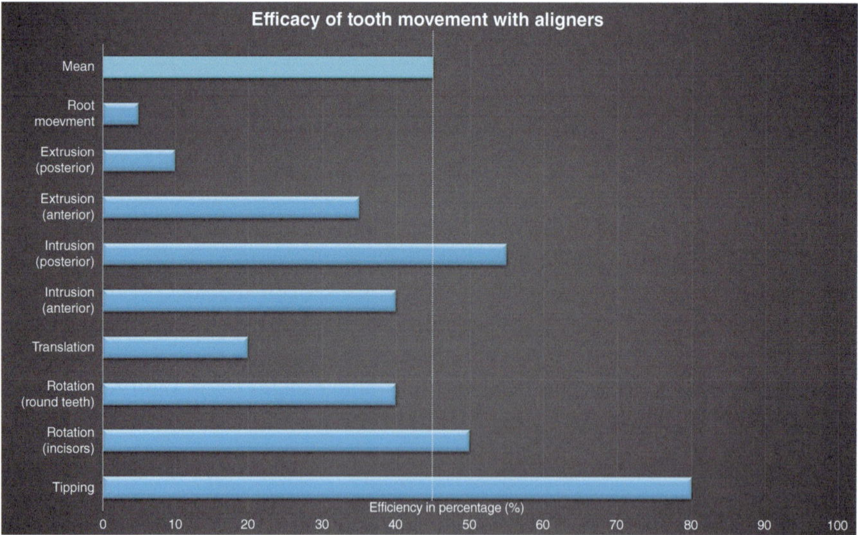

Fig. 4.14 The mean efficacy of tooth movements achieved with aligners. This diagram has been obtained from the Journal of the World Federation of Orthodontists, 2022, and the permission kindly provided by Elsevier

4.5.3 Virtual C-Chain

Virtual c-chain can be prescribed in cases with excessive interdental spacing at the end of the active treatment. This is usually due to excessive IPR or irreversible distortion of contact points at points where IPR has been undertaken. The virtual c-chain can be prescribed in the overcorrection stage.

It is prudent to follow-up the patients when virtual c-chains are applied as overclosure could cause intrusion of the teeth onto which it is prescribed. It is thus contraindicated in the following cases:

1. Absence of interdental spacing.
2. Abnormal interdental contact points.
3. Lack of maxillary incisor protrusion with no scope of lingual tipping.
4. Lack of mandibular incisor proclination with no scope of lingual tipping.
5. Existing favourable interincisor angle.

4.6 Tray Trimming

Finishing can be one of the most difficult stages of the treatment. One of the frequent causes behind this difficulty is the lack of precise fit between the aligner and tooth surface.

Trays can be trimmed with scissors, burs, altered with flaps, or have cut-outs obtained with hand pliers.

One of the areas, which is affected by this more than others, is the upper lateral incisor region. This is also an area which exhibits more tracking issues than others. Figure 4.15 below illustrates a technique to improve the fit of the aligner over the upper lateral incisor. The tray is trimmed on the palatal aspect of this tooth in a "U-shape" to enable the engagement of an elastic band. A button cut-out for the placement of a composite button should be placed on the gingival aspect of this

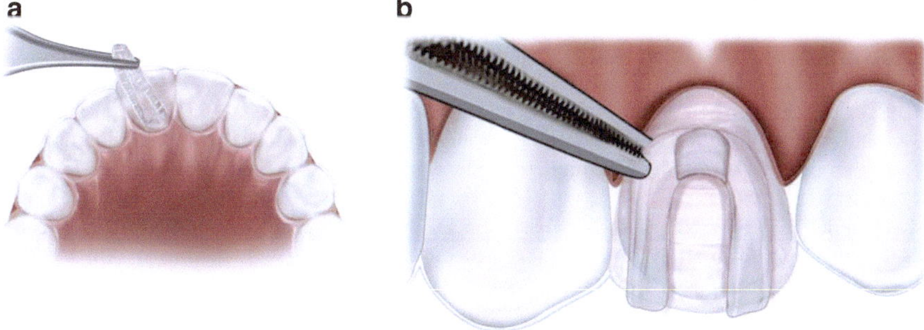

Fig. 4.15 (**a**) occlusal view (**b**) buccal view illustrating a clinical technique to improve aligner fit over the incisal surface of a tooth. This is indicated for cases exhibiting difficulties in finishing due to poor adaptation of the aligner over the tooth surface

tooth and the elastic band is pulled from the buccal aspect over to the palatal aspect allowing an intrusive force to act on the aligner and improve its fitting over the incisor edge of the tooth. This technique can be applied to other teeth that pose a similar difficulty.

In cases where button cut-outs need to be introduced following the order of the active trays, the clinician can introduce these by using a cut-out plier or by using a bur to allow space for the introduction of the composite button. This allows both the clinician and the patient to progress with the intended trays and avoid waiting for the fabrication and shipping of a new batch of refinement aligners.

References

1. Condo R, Pazzini L, Cerroni L, Pasquantonio G, Lagana G, Pecora A, et al. Mechanical properties of "two generations" of teeth aligners: change analysis during oral permanence. Dent Mater J. 2018;37(5):835–42.
2. Condo R, Mampieri G, Giancotti A, Cerroni L, Pasquantonio G, Divizia A, et al. SEM characterization and ageing analysis on two generation of invisible aligners. BMC Oral Health. 2021;21(1):316.
3. Bakdach WMM, Haiba M, Hadad R. Changes in surface morphology, chemical and mechanical properties of clear aligners during intraoral usage: a systematic review and meta-analysis. Int Orthod. 2022;20(1):100610.
4. Bruno GGA, Barone M, Mutinelli S, De Stefani A. Invisalign® vs. SparkTM template: which is the most effective in the attachment bonding procedure? A randomized controlled trial. Appl Sci. 2021;11(15):1–6.
5. Mantovani E, Castroflorio E, Rossini G, Garino F, Cugliari G, Deregibus A, et al. Scanning electron microscopy analysis of aligner fitting on anchorage attachments. J Orofac Orthop. 2019;80(2):79–87.
6. Mantovani E, Castroflorio E, Rossini G, Garino F, Cugliari G, Deregibus A, et al. Scanning electron microscopy evaluation of aligner fit on teeth. Angle Orthod. 2018;88(5):596–601.
7. Lombardo L, Palone M, Longo M, Arveda N, Nacucchi M, De Pascalis F, et al. MicroCT X-ray comparison of aligner gap and thickness of six brands of aligners: an in-vitro study. Prog Orthod. 2020;21(1):12.
8. Ryokawa H, Miyazaki Y, Fujishima A, Miyazaki T, Maki K. The mechanical properties of dental thermoplastic materials in a simulated intraoral environment. Orthod Waves. 2006;65(2):64–72.
9. Lombardo L, Martines E, Mazzanti V, Arreghini A, Mollica F, Siciliani G. Stress relaxation properties of four orthodontic aligner materials: a 24-hour in vitro study. Angle Orthod. 2017;87(1):11–8.
10. Palone M, Longo M, Arveda N, Nacucchi M, Pascalis F, Spedicato GA, et al. Micro-computed tomography evaluation of general trends in aligner thickness and gap width after thermoforming procedures involving six commercial clear aligners: an in vitro study. Korean J Orthod. 2021;51(2):135–41.
11. Haouili N, Kravitz ND, Vaid NR, Ferguson DJ, Makki L. Has Invisalign improved? A prospective follow-up study on the efficacy of tooth movement with Invisalign. Am J Orthod Dentofacial Orthop. 2020;158(3):420–5.
12. Sachdev S, Tantidhnazet S, Saengfai NN. Accuracy of tooth movement with in-house clear aligners. J World Fed Orthod. 2021;10(4):177–82.
13. Upadhyay M, Arqub SA. Biomechanics of clear aligners: hidden truths & first principles. J World Fed Orthod. 2022;11(1):12–21.

Part II

Clinical Management of Malocclusions

Navigating Through the Software   5

5.1   Introduction

The full potential of the Invisalign® system and its accompanying software can be exploited by the clinician if an extensive knowledge of its features is acquired at the very start of adopting this technique. Familiarisation with each individual step and methodological use of the software stages ensures a more realistic outcome in line with the digital projection.

This chapter focuses on the processes that follow collection of records discussed in detail in Chap. 3.

5.2   The Patients' Online Folder

The clinical team involved in a patient's treatment will have access to the patient's folder. Each folder will in turn have the details input on submission including patient's details, type of treatment allocated, records placed, and the ordering stage.

The clinical team will at this stage have the possibility of placing an order for

- Additional aligners
- Replacement aligners
- Attachment templates
- Vivera retainers
- Starting a new treatment

In the "Recent Documents" section, the clinical has access to;

- The prescription form submitted
- The ClinCheck Plan
- The treatment overview

© The Author(s), under exclusive license to Springer Nature Switzerland AG 2024   51
S. Abela, *Aligner Systems in Invisible Orthodontics*,
https://doi.org/10.1007/978-3-031-49204-4_5

– Clinical photographs
– Order confirmation

The additional service section of a patient's folder will allow:

– Generation of an aligner schedule
– Scheduling of appointments
– Transfer of a patient to another Invisalign provider
– Cancellation of the order
– Sharing the ClinCheck plan

One additional section is the access to the shipping labels and form for couriering and dispatching services.

5.3 The Patients' ClinCheck Plan

The ClinCheck Pro® 6 is a proprietary software enabling the digital visualisation and digital manipulation of a virtual 3D model set-up to a digital prescription. This digital prescription will ultimately result in the manufacturing of a batch of active orthodontic aligners. It also enables a stage-by-stage representation of the individual and collective tooth movements to provide a rendering of the real-world progress from start to finish.

The software has an easy-to-follow page layout with two taskbars on the top of the page and a treatment plan section on the right-hand side of the screen. The bottom part of the page allows the clinical staff member to return to the original set-up prior to any modifications carried out.

The uppermost task bar has four tabs:

1. Return to the Invisalign ClinCheck Pro® 6 doctor's site
2. The patient's details with a drop-down menu that displays three sections:
    (a) Section 1. Listing the category of patient based on age
    (b) Section 2. The facility of
        (i) Exporting the 3D simulation in a movie, screenshot or STL formats
        (ii) Sharing the ClinCheck® plan via email
        (iii) looking at the treatment overview
    (c) Section 3. This section displays two user options: "Other actions" tab which refers to the possibility of switching the level of treatment provision or cancelling the order or hiding the patient's information from the task bar
3. The "Notes" tab is a section where both the user and the company's technicians can leave to describe further details about the case
4. The doctor's details

The second task bar has all the features that enable the clinician to change, alter, modify and set the models on display. The features displayed from left to right of the screen are as follows:

- "RECs" icon enables visualisation of the records available to the user.
- "Zoom" icon enables zooming in or out to improve visualisation of the digitised models.
- "Rotate" icon enables rotation of the models.
- "Pan" icon enables the vertical manipulation of the models.
- "Upper" icon enables visualisation of the upper arch in isolation.
- "Maxil" icon enables occlusal view of the upper arch in isolation.
- "Right" icon enables visualisation of the right-hand side of the set-up models.
- "Anter" icon enables visualisation of the anterior aspect of the set-up models.
- "Left" icon enables visualisation of the left-hand side of the set-up models.
- "Mand" icon enables occlusal view of the lower arch in isolation.
- "Lower" icon enables visualisation of the lower arch in isolation.
- "Comp" icon enables the right, anterior, left sides and upper and lower occlusal aspects of the arches to be visualised.
- "Smile" icon enables software prediction of the patient's smile after uploading the patient's extraoral smiling photo using the Invisalign Photo Uploader.
- "Super" icon enables the superimposition of the different treatment stages over the initial presentation.
- "Grid" enables the use of the measurement grid where each square is 10 mm by 10 mm with each box within the grid being further divided into 1 mm squares.
- "Attach" icon enables the visualisation of additional aligner features such as attachments, precision cuts and bite ramps amongst others. A blue-coloured line beneath this icon indicates the presence of one of these features present for the case being modified on the software.
- "Occlus" icon enables the visualisation of heavy inter arch contacts with green-coloured tooth surfaces of teeth indicate light contact spots whilst red-coloured tooth surfaces indicate heavy inter arch occlusal contacts. The former and latter are represented by respectively coloured dots next to the icon.
- "IPR" icon enables the visualisation of interproximal reduction instructions or spacing presented in the plan being viewed on the ClinCheck Pro® 6 software.
- "Staging" icon enables the visualisation of the tooth movement staging for each tooth and for each arch. Bite correction stages and overcorrection stages can also be visualised by clicking on the icon
- "Tables" icon enables the visualisation of the tooth movement types for each tooth and for each arch. This is available for both coronal and radicular movements. The movements included are: extrusion and intrusion movements, relative extrusion and intrusion movements, buccal or lingual translation in mms, mesial or distal translation in mms, rotational, angular and inclination movement in degrees.

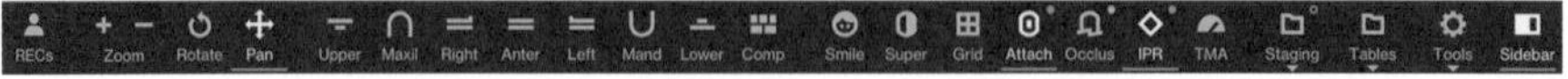

Fig. 5.1 Diagrammatic representation of the icons in the second task bar. This figure has been reproduced from ClinCheck Pro 6® software and reproduced by kind permission of Align Technology, Inc. (Santa Clara, Calif., USA)

This icon also holds the Bolton analysis for the case with the dentoalveolar excess region highlighted and specified. This is done for the intercanine and the intermolar region. This excess can be in mms or in percentages. The individual tooth dimensions are also specified.

This icon also holds the arch width dimensions in the intercanine, interpremolar, and the intermolar and the differences between the start and end of treatment.

This icon also holds the overjet (OJ) and overbite (OB) values including the pre- and post-treatment difference in values. The values are represented in mms.

This icon holds the tooth numbering feature which when activated will appear on the tooth surfaces.

- "Tools" icon represents additional features of the ClinCheck Pro® that can be explored by the user and the possibility of customising the number of icons that can be seen on the taskbar.

The additional features include tooth movement assessments, pontics, eruption compensation and occlusal plane inclination.

The sidebar feature showing the current treatment plan and the past treatment plans can be activated or deactivated by collapsing it to increase the operating window size.

All the above icons are diagrammatically presented in Fig. 5.1 below:

5.4 Modifying the Patients' ClinCheck® Plan

Once the user opts to modify the plan, the "New Modification" tab will need to be activated. The second section "Comment to The Tech" together with the "New Modification" tab are present on the right-hand side of the user window.

In the "New Modification" section, the user has two features that can further modify the existing set-up:

- "Movements"—This includes "Tooth", "Features" and "Arch" for modification of the individual tooth movements, inclusion of features and arch modification, respectively.
- "IPR"—This includes three options for the user to choose from: "Auto," "Maintain" and "No IPR" for automatic inclusion of IPR by the software, maintaining the exist level of IPR and exclusion of IPR.

These settings are better illustrated in Fig. 5.2 below.

Fig. 5.2 Diagrammatic representation of "Tooth," "Features" and "Arch" sections for both the "Movements" and "IPR" sections on the ClinCheck® Pro 6. This figure has been reproduced from ClinCheck Pro 6® software and reproduced by kind permission of Align Technology, Inc. (Santa Clara, Calif., USA)

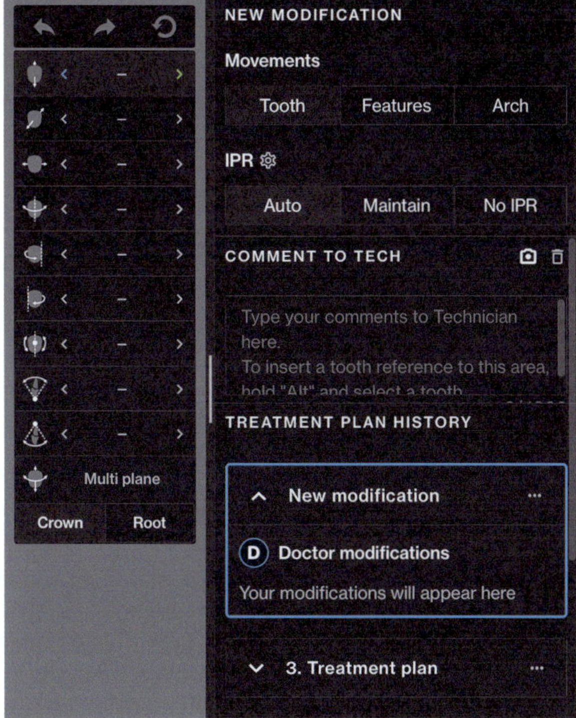

The user can place suggestions for further improvements to the set-up. The "Comment To Tech" section includes two icons one representing a camera enabling the user to take a snapshot of the current 3D model set-up to explain the tooth movement needed better and one delete function represented with a trash icon.

ClinCheck Pro® Live Update for 3D controls is the latest update on the ClinCheck Pro® software which allows live updating of the model set-up once the user has completed and placed the final instructions and modifications.

5.5   Options for Modifying the Patients' ClinCheck Plan

The user classically enters the user interface of the software to access the model set-up and tailor the plan to the patient. The user has numerous opportunities to modify the plan on the software. At each opportunity, the user is faced with four decision possibilities:

1. The user could opt to resolve the difficulty being faced with the model set-up presented with.
2. The user can switch plans, for example, from an Invisalign Lite Plan to an Invisalign Comprehensive plan.

3. The user can decide to delete the plan altogether due to the non-feasibility nature of the proposed plan.
4. The user can decide to continue with the modifications and produce further plans for future consideration.

5.6   New Features Available on the ClinCheck Pro® 6.0

5.6.1   Red Zones

A new feature that has been introduced with the latest version of the software includes the addition of red zones with a new attachment placement.

This helps the user identify areas of the teeth where the placement of an attachment is not possible. The doctor will be notified via the Live Update.

5.6.2   ClinCheck Live Update

An additional new feature is the ClinCheck Live Update which enables the user to activate and will have the new plan presented live. This is valid for the 3D controls and the main aim of this introduction is to hasten the modifications of treatment plans on the software and expedite production of the final aligners.

5.6.3   In-Face Visualisation Feature

An additional new feature includes the in-face visualisation feature. This is the software anticipatory visualisation of the patient's new smile and fitted to the smiling extraoral photo. This helps give the patient the overall enhancement of their smile following treatment.

Clinical Management of Class I Cases

6

6.1 Introduction

This chapter focuses on the processes that need to be followed for a successful treatment of class I malocclusions.

The following descriptions and terminologies are commonly associated with this type of malocclusion.

Definition: The mandibular incisor edges lie or are below the cingulum plateau of the maxillary incisors [1].

Incidence: 60–70% of all malocclusions.

Extraoral features:

– Straight profile

Soft tissue features:

– Competent/incompetent lips
– Normal/deep/shallow labio-mental sulcus

Intraoral features:

– Incisor relationship: Class I incisor relationship
– Canine relationship: The mesial incline of the upper canine overlaps the distal slope of the lower canine (the maxillary canine occludes between the mandibular canine and the first premolar)
– Molar relationship: The mesio-buccal cusp of the maxillary first permanent molar occludes in the anterior-buccal groove of the mandibular first permanent molar

© The Author(s), under exclusive license to Springer Nature Switzerland AG 2024
S. Abela, *Aligner Systems in Invisible Orthodontics*,
https://doi.org/10.1007/978-3-031-49204-4_6

6.2   Align Technology Grading of Case Difficulty

Align Technology, Inc. method of grading class I malocclusions is identical to grading of any other type of aligner cases. Classification of class I cases are mostly based on the degree of crowding and are as follows:

Mild/simple class I

– Colour code: green
– Dental extractions: none
– Distalisation: less than 2 mm
– Crowding per arch: less than 6 mm
– Expansion per quadrant: less than 2 mm

Moderate/intermediate class I

– Colour code: blue
– Dental extractions: none
– Distalisation: between 2 and 4 mm
– Crowding per arch: between 6 and 8 mm
– Expansion per quadrant: between 2 and 4 mm

Severe/complex class I

– Colour code: black
– Dental extractions: yes
– Distalisation: more than 4 mm
– Crowding per arch: more than 8 mm
– Expansion per quadrant: more than 4 mm

In the mildest form, the case is more predictable with less complex movements involved and less than 2 mm individual tooth movements.

For moderate cases, the predictability is more variable with individual tooth movements of between 2 and 4 mm whilst for more complex cases, the predictability is more uncertain with movements potentially exceeding 4 mm.

The software can make allowances for the anticipations with A-P correction using class II elastics with a "virtual jump".

6.3   Predicting Treatment Outcomes

The predictability of class I cases depend on two major factors: the degree of crowding or spacing present and the degree of arch constriction.

It is more predictable if a patient with a class I malocclusion presents with the following:

– In an active phase of growth
– A high potential for expansion of the arch
– A degree of tooth retroclination especially in the labial segment region
– A degree of palatal crown tipping in the buccal segments
– Class I buccal segment relationship
– Class I canine relationship

Predictability of dental closure for cases that present with interdental spacing is improved if the following features are present:

– Opposing arch lengths and sizes match
– Good arch shape and form
– Acceptable crown morphology
– Spacing present due to labial segment proclination

6.4 Formulating the Treatment Plan

At the prescription stage of the treatment, the treating clinician has two important aspects of the malocclusion to determine:

1. The amount and type of attachments needed
2. The degree of proclination that is permissible in the labial regions

The clinician has several design options that can be embedded in the aligner design to improve the clinical outcomes in class I cases. These are listed below in chronological order of preference and clinical ease of use:

1. Conventional or optimised attachments or a combination of both
2. IPR in the labial or buccal segments or both
3. Labial segment proclination
4. Buccal segment expansion
5. Buccal segment distalisation
6. Orthodontic mini-implants (OMIs) or temporary anchorage devices (TADS)—supported mesialising or distalising appliances
7. Dental extractions
8. Surgical correction

6.4.1 Optimised Attachments

Attachments as well as conventional in shape and design can also be optimised to provide the ideal forces with the aligner and the attachment interaction. Planned inclusion of attachments or acceptance of the default set-up provided by the software's algorithms is now considered synonymous with aligner provision. Align

Technology, Inc. proprietary optimised attachments have been questioned with regard to their efficiency when compared to conventional composite attachments [2]. Attachment size, shape, number and position on a tooth surface can be changed and configured as best possible for the intended moment; however, it has also been observed that the size or shape or an attachment has minimal bearing if at all on bodily tooth movement [3]. Although aesthetically attachments might represent a compromise their loss is associated with a decreased aligners' effectiveness [4].

Attachments can be optimised as follows:

1. Optimised rotation attachments: These attachments are shaped with a bevel towards the side of the tooth where the de-rotational movement is needed. The aligner buccal and lingual interface with these types of attachments will result in a de-rotational movement. These are usually placed on upper and lower premolars and canines.
2. Multi-plane attachments: These attachments are shaped to provide a force in multi-directional planes. Lingual attachments will also assist with this type of movement. The same attachment will allow different trays to move a tooth in different planes at different stages of the treatment. These are usually placed on upper lateral incisors.
3. Occlusal attachments: These types of attachments are normally indicated in cases with short clinical crowns to increase retention of the aligner.
4. Optimised root attachments: These attachments are designed with the bevel on the side to which the root needs to move. These attachments are also designed in a vertical manner to provide more contact surface area or as a complementary set of two on the same tooth surface. These are usually placed on upper central and lateral incisors and upper and lower canines and premolars.

6.4.2 IPR

The main indications for IPR can be the following:

1. Tooth-size discrepancies

    In instances where cases present with tooth-size discrepancies, the crown proportions between the upper and lower teeth are mismatched. The deviation from the average crown widths can be visualised. Wider teeth than the average can be reduced with IPR. Alternatively, diminutive teeth can be widened prosthetically. If the tooth-size discrepancies are too large to correct with IPR or prosthetic camouflage, the treatment plan would need to include additional measures to address this.

    The best methodology to identify tooth-size discrepancies is to use the Bolton's formula. This formula obtains the ratio of tooth sizes between:
    (a) The upper and lower labial segments from the distal aspects of the canines
    (b) The upper and lower buccal and labial segments from the distal aspect of the first molars

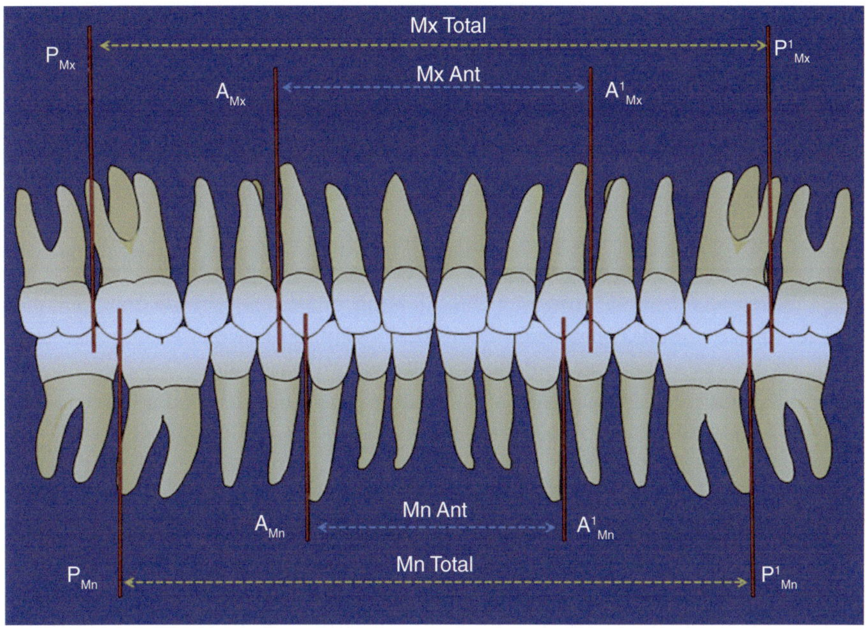

Fig. 6.1 The Bolton's analysis of tooth-size discrepancies where the ratio of the mesio-distal widths of the crowns between the two arches is measured. This could be measured for the labial segments or for both labial and buccal segments. (This figure was reproduced from Am J Orthod Dentofacial Orthop 2013;143:574–85, with kind permission of Elsevier)

Calculating these two ratios is done by simplistically measuring the mesio-distal widths of the teeth in the labial segment and obtaining the percentage of lower relative to upper.

The arithmetic division of the two total mesio-distal widths should equate to 77.2 with a range of ±1.65.

In case of wanting to identify any discrepancies in the whole arch the mesio-distal widths of the lower arch from the first molar to the contralateral molar is proportioned to those in the upper arch. In this case the ration should equate to 91.3 with a range of ±1.91. Figure 6.1 below illustrates this concept for the anterior segments and for the whole arch.

The ability to obtain these figures is a clear indication to the clinician that it is possible to obtain a class I occlusion with average features in occlusion.

Should the ratios be outside the range of deviation formalised by Bolton in 1958, the presence of tooth-size discrepancies may manifest in deviations from a class I occlusion within the upper or lower arch depending on the localisation of the discrepancy [5].

For example, in cases of excessive tooth widths in the upper arch with well-aligned dentition in the lower arch, the occlusion would feature an increased overjet. In cases of excessive widths affecting the mandibular teeth that are also in good alignment, the upper dentition will be spaced to accommodate the increased mesio-distal arch width of the lower arch.

Identification of Bolton's tooth-size discrepancies is the main reason that IPR is prescribed together with elimination of crowding to secure a non-extraction approach [6].

2. Mild to moderate crowding

The classification of crowding, based on the amount of crowding present can be described as follows:

- Mild crowding with space requirements of up to 4 mm
- Moderate crowding with space requirements of between 5 and 8 mm
- Severe with space requirements of greater than 8 mm

Based on the above crowding classification, clinicians vary the treatment plan accordingly. Should space gain be needed solely to relieve crowding. Table 6.1 below provides classical guidelines for this approach.

IPR is ideally suited for cases that have crowding of less than 6 mm. This would constitute cases that present with mild and/or moderate crowding. Cases presenting with moderate and/or severe crowding constitute the need for an extraction approach, and IPR has recently put this into question. Several studies have described the amount of crowding that IPR can relieve. On the upper limits relieve of up to 10 mm on premolars and molars only and 13 mm between the second molar in the mandible have been described [7].

Using Table 6.2 below as a reference and using the means of interproximal enamel thicknesses for the maxillary and mandibular dentition, the maximum space gains possible by IPR are 13.40 mm and 10.98 mm, respectively.

Table 6.1 Recommended treatment approaches, based on the amount of crowding present

Degree of crowding	Extraction approach	Additional treatment approaches
Mild crowding (up to 4 mm)	Non-extraction	• IPR • Lower incisor proclination • Buccal distalisation • Maxillary transverse expansion

Moderate crowding (5–6 mm)	• Non-extraction
	• Extraction
	  – Single: Lower incisor
	  – Multiple: Second premolars
		• IPR
		• Lower incisor proclination
		• Buccal distalisation
		• Maxillary transverse expansion

Moderate crowding (7–8 mm)	Extraction
	  – Multiple: First premolars
	  – Multiple: Second premolars
		• IPR
		• Lower incisor proclination
		• Buccal distalisation
		• Maxillary transverse expansion

Severe crowding (greater than 8 mm)	Extraction – Multiple: First premolars	• IPR • Lower incisor proclination • Buccal distalisation • Maxillary transverse expansion

Table 6.2 Mesial and distal interproximal enamel thickness for each tooth for both maxillary and mandibular arches (adapted from Hershkovitz, 2015 [8])

	PET medial aspect in mm	PET distal aspect in mm	Proximal enamel thickness mean in mm
Maxillary dentition			
Central incisor	0.81 ± 0.06	0.81 ± 0.27	0.81
Lateral incisor	0.76 ± 0.14	0.86 ± 0.28	0.81
Canine	1.10 ± 0.21	1.11 ± 0.26	1.10
First premolar	1.13 ± 0.15	1.25 ± 0.37	1.19
Second premolar	1.41 ± 0.27	1.36 ± 0.30	1.38
First molar	1.35 ± 0.29	1.48 ± 0.17	1.41
Mandibular dentition			
Central and lateral incisors	0.64 ± 0.19	0.60 ± 0.18	0.62
Canine	0.97 ± 0.21	1.30 ± 0.61	1.13
First premolar	1.16 ± 0.13	1.05 ± 0.24	1.10
Second premolar	1.23 ± 0.10	1.30 ± 0.20	1.26
First molar	1.37 ± 0.12	1.40 ± 0.20	1.38

3. Improving contact points

   Improving the contact points between teeth, by contouring the interproximal sides of teeth also addresses the aesthetic aspect. This is even more relevant in the presence of misshapen teeth, upper incisors with and more triangular-shaped teeth.

4. Reduction in size of gingival embrasures

   Interproximal reduction lengthens the contact point areas between teeth leading to a reduction in the gingival embrasures also referred to as "black triangles", the unfilled space between gingival papillae between the alveolar crest and the dental contact points. It has been estimated that optimal gingival embrasure aesthetics is present when this distance is less than 5 mm [9, 10].

5. Improved long-term stability

   IPR as a modality to increase long-term stability has been contested for a very long time. Weak associations have been drawn between IPR, reduction of tooth size and prevention of increase in intercanine width and relapse [11, 12]. In previous studies, IPR has also been investigated in conjunction with circumferential supracrestal fiberotomy (CSF); however, this technique is not practised frequently nowadays [13, 14].

   Contraindications for IPR include the following:

1. Severe rotations with displaced contact points
2. Unstable periodontal disease
3. Heavily restored dentition with mesial and distal restorations
4. Moderate to severe crowding
5. Generalised sensitivity
6. Increased pulp to crown ratios
7. High caries risk

Methods of providing IPR can include hand-held diamond strips which in turn can be single or double-sided and of various sizes. As the strip is placed interdentally, the size would be in relation to the height of the crown which is being trimmed. Contra-angle handpieces with oscillating strips can be used as well as air rotor stripping with discs or with burs.

In general, clinicians tend to provide less IPR than the amount prescribed during the planning stages; however, the use of air rotor handpieces provides the most IPR when compared to other techniques. The use of gauges to assess the amount of IPR delivered is recommended [15].

The IPR technique is deemed to be safe and the use of desensitising gel or toothpaste following the procedure lessens the incidence of postoperative discomfort, increased sensitivity and rise of new carious lesions [16].

6.4.2.1 Interproximal Enamel Thickness

Interproximal reduction, IPR has become a mainstream technique used very frequently and closely associated with clear aligner therapy. IPR might also be referred to as enamel stripping, trimming, slandering or reproximation. Knowledge of the enamel thickness is key in providing this technique successfully. The proximal thickness is usually very similar between the right and left sides; however, it varies significantly between individuals and also between labial and buccal segments. The mesio-distal widths is also very different between genders with males having larger mesio-distal crown widths mostly due to larger proportions of dentine in comparison to enamel in females [7]. In general, the enamel thickness on the distal aspect of teeth surpasses the mesial enamel thickness. This is usually observed throughout the entirety of the upper and lower arches by 0.1 mm [17]. Table 6.2 below tabulates the interproximal enamel thickness for each tooth. The figures might vary between different studies. Both mesial and distal aspects of each tooth are outlined below.

6.4.2.2 Safe Margins for Interproximal Enamel Reduction

Every clinician, based on the above facts, will need to provide a prescription for the inclusion and amount of IPR needed for each individual case. Variations have been clearly identified earlier with gender differences, variation between mesial and distal aspects of teeth and between the two arches being the norm. Gender variation has also been reported in the past with African-Americans having thicker interproximal enamel thickness than Caucasians [10].

A specific investigation of enamel thickness variation within the mandibular arch by Hall et al., 2007 concluded that in the lower labial segment it is safe practice to perform 0.2 mm of IPR. This was in line with a histological study by Sarig et al. (2015) concluding that 0.25 and 0.5 mm of IPR per surface in the labial and buccal segments was safe practice [8]. This could be extended to 0.3 mm per surface in the canine region. Table 6.3 below tabulates the safe amount of IPR that can be carried out in both arches.

Long-term harmful effects of IPR have been excluded in previously conducted studies. Risks of increased enamel surface roughness post-IPR can be eliminated by

Table 6.3 Safe amount of IPR per tooth surface and per contact area

Safe margins for IPR		
	Amount of IPR per surface in mm	Amount of IPR per contact area in mm
Maxillary and mandibular dentition		
Central incisor	0.25	0.5
Lateral incisor	0.25	0.5
Canine	0.3	0.6
First premolar	0.5	1.0
Second premolar	0.5	1.0
First molar	0.5	1

careful polishing. The latter would also eliminate the possibility of increased risk of plaque accumulation and carious lesions developing. Approximating roots was also shown to be safe with no long-term risks to the periodontium. Vigorous use of the IPR technique can however irreversibly damage the contact points and prevent full post orthodontic closure of the interdental areas and can also lead to soft tissue trauma.

6.4.3   Labial Segment Proclination

One of the methods of gaining space within an arch is to procline the teeth within the labial segments. In fixed appliance therapy, usually this takes place in the initial phases of treatment. The indications in clear therapy include lingually tipped incisors or crowding. During the proclination stages, the incisors and canines are tipped buccally leading to a change in the occlusal plane, relative intrusion and reduction in the overbite. The limits of proclination should be based on the amount of crowding present in addition to the other aspects of the prescription that will be addressing the occlusal features.

6.4.4   Arch Expansion

The clinician prescribing the treatment has a multitude of options that can enable arch expansion. This applies for expansion in the canine to the most posterior molars. The clinician can specify these for every case by enlisting them in the clinical preference section or tailoring them per case. The expansion sites can be specified as follows:

- In the intercanine and premolar region only
- In the molar region only
- In the premolar and molar region only
- A combination of the above involving expansion in the canine, premolar and molar region
- Maintenance of the arch shape and width without expansion

The magnitude of expansion can also be specified as it being less or equal than 2 mm or more than 2 mm per quadrant. Measurements of the expansion obtained is usually taken at three points in the arch; intercanine cusp tips, mid-point of buccal cusp tip of the first or second premolar and the mid-point of the mesio-buccal cusp tip of the first molar. Equivalent palatal points can also be taken as reference points. In past studies, Invisalign® aligners were found to be effective at providing a certain degree of expansion, achieved mostly by tipping movements. No bodily movement was noticed [18]. Similar findings were observed in a study analysing the accuracy of the ClinCheck's® predictability of the final outcome [19]. Most of the expansion movement was also seen to be obtained by tipping movements. The maxillary premolar region exhibited the greatest amount of expansion with an average of +5.2° to +6.9° whilst the molar region averaged 4°. The region that exhibited the least predictable expansion was the canine region. In a separate study analysing the benefits of Invisalign® First system for maxillary expansion in mixed dentitions, the advantages over traditional removable appliances were evident [20]. Measurements and comparisons were obtained from digital study models superimposition.

6.4.5 Buccal Segment Distalisation

The intention of resorting to buccal segment distalisation is twofold; lengthening the arch for space gains and alteration of buccal segment relationships. This movement with clear aligner therapy and more specifically with Invisalign® is a very predictable movement. The actuation of the process is favourable as anchorage is obtained from all the labial segment and premolar regions reinforcing anchorage positively. A study has also proven the efficiency of this type of tooth movement together with the possibility of actuating bodily movement of the molars. A distalisation of 2.25 mm was observed with the use of vertical attachments without tipping nor vertical movements [21].

6.4.6 TADS-Supported Mesialising or Distalising Appliances

Orthodontic mini-implants (OMIs) also referred to as orthodontic mini-screws or temporary anchorage devices (TADS) have provided a very ubiquitous influence in orthodontics, and this is no different with treatment involving clear aligners.

Several clinicians, case reports and scientific articles are available documenting the use of these anchorage devices.

A full description of their adjunctive use in clear aligner therapy is found in Chap. 13.

6.4.7 Dental Extractions

With cases needing dental extractions, the treating clinician has to ensure that several steps in the prescription are undertaken to ensure optimal outcomes.

Power arms (PAs) inclusion in the prescription allows the inclusion of cut-outs to be included for manual placement of these auxiliary items. Align Technology, Inc. calls these design features a convenience feature, and it can be prescribed on any tooth.

- Lower incisor extraction
- Cases being treated with lower incisor extraction; the attachment protocol has to change to include vertical attachments on either side of the extraction site to prevent excessive tipping of the incisors distal to the extraction zone. These are 1 mm thick and are automatically included by the software unless optimised attachments are set by default.
- Premolar extraction
- The attachment protocol for premolar extractions needs to ensure distal root tipping of the tooth mesial to the extraction site whilst the opposite is valid for the root of the tooth distal to the extraction site.

The attachment protocol also needs to ensure that the attachments serve to anchor the teeth as a unit distal to the extraction site if the incisors need to be retracted. The default setting by the in-built Artificial Intelligence (AI) of the ClinCheck® pre-sets the staging of the tooth movement with two thirds of the movement focused on labial segment retraction whilst the rest, one third focused on posterior segment mesialisation. This is also totally customisable by the treating clinician.

6.4.8   Surgical Correction

The use of clear aligners is nowadays so widespread that it can also be considered for orthodontic malocclusions requiring orthognathic surgery.

Given the contemporaneous nature of the appliances, their utilisation to treat surgical cases could be unfamiliar for the whole team, orthodontic and oral surgeon specialists alike. The push from patients to have more discrete appliances given the lengthy nature of the treatment has led to the exploration of this modality.

Further details on treating orthognathic cases with clear aligners is found in Chap. 12.

6.5   Features of a Class I Malocclusion to Be Given Special Consideration

6.5.1   Interdental Spacing

Interdental spacing could be the only feature that a patient with a class I malocclusion presents with.

This could be due to the following:

- A tooth-size discrepancy within one arch or between the two arches: In the former case, the opposing arch would have well aligned teeth and the treatment solutions could either be space redistribution or prosthetic camouflage. In the latter case, the opposing arch would feature dental crowding, and this would need to be addressed prior to addressing the interdental spacing in the affected arch.

- Proclination of the labial segment: Closure of these spaces will result in lingual or palatal crown tipping with relative extrusion which would in turn result in an increase in overbite. Long-term retention will be needed in these cases long term to ensure stability and prevent relapse.
- Diminutive or peg-shaped teeth: Diminutive teeth can be generalised in one arch or in both arches; however, it most commonly affects upper lateral incisors. The treatment solution as for tooth-size discrepancies consists of redistributing spaces such as localising the spacing distal to the upper lateral incisors, IPR in the opposing arch to decrease the arch length of the opposing arch or prosthetic camouflage.
- Hypodontia: Missing teeth can be the cause of spacing. Most commonly affected regions are upper and lower premolar regions, upper lateral incisor regions and lower incisor regions.

6.5.2 Open Bite

With class I malocclusions presenting with open bite, they will invariably need extrusions of single teeth or multiple teeth.

Single tooth attachments or numerous teeth attachments will be needed for single or multiple teeth, respectively. In the latter's case, the teeth in the buccal segment will be intruded to allow a greater correctional effect on the open bite closure. The attachments deliver 0.5 mm of extrusion.

The clinician can opt to have one of the following strategies to address an anterior open bite:

- Extrude upper incisors only
- Extrude upper incisors and intrude buccal segments in the upper arch or lower arch or in both
- Surgical correction

References

1. British Standards Institute. Glossary of dental terms (BS 4492). London: BSI; 1983.
2. Karras T, Singh M, Karkazis E, Liu D, Nimeri G, Ahuja B. Efficacy of Invisalign attachments: a retrospective study. Am J Orthod Dentofacial Orthop. 2021;160(2):250–8.
3. Ho CT, Huang YT, Chao CW, Huang TH, Kao CT. Effects of different aligner materials and attachments on orthodontic behavior. J Dent Sci. 2021;16(3):1001–9.
4. Yaosen C, Mohamed AM, Jinbo W, Ziwei Z, Al-Balaa M, Yan Y. Risk factors of composite attachment loss in orthodontic patients during orthodontic clear aligner therapy: a prospective study. Biomed Res Int. 2021;2021:6620377.

5. Bolton WA. Disharmony in tooth size and its relation to the analysis and treatment of malocclusion*. Angle Orthod. 1958;28(3):113–30.

6. Lapenaite E, Lopatiene K. Interproximal enamel reduction as a part of orthodontic treatment. Stomatologija. 2014;16(1):19–24.

7. Stroud JL, English J, Buschang PH. Enamel thickness of the posterior dentition: its implications for nonextraction treatment. Angle Orthod. 1998;68(2):141–6.

8. Sarig R, Vardimon AD, Sussan C, Benny L, Sarne O, Hershkovitz I, et al. Pattern of maxillary and mandibular proximal enamel thickness at the contact area of the permanent dentition from first molar to first molar. Am J Orthod Dentofacial Orthop. 2015;147(4):435–44.

9. Tarnow DP, Magner AW, Fletcher P. The effect of the distance from the contact point to the crest of bone on the presence or absence of the interproximal dental papilla. J Periodontol. 1992;63(12):995–6.

10. Meredith L, Mei L, Cannon RD, Farella M. Interproximal reduction in orthodontics: why, where, how much to remove? Aust Orthod J. 2017;33(2):150–7.

11. Peck H, Peck S. An index for assessing tooth shape deviations as applied to the mandibular incisors. Am J Orthod. 1972;61(4):384–401.

12. Gilmore CA, Little RM. Mandibular incisor dimensions and crowding. Am J Orthod. 1984;86(6):493–502.

13. Boese LR. Fiberotomy and reproximation without lower retention, nine years in retrospect: part I. Angle Orthod. 1980;50(2):88–97.

14. Boese LR. Fiberotomy and reproximation without lower retention 9 years in retrospect: part II. Angle Orthod. 1980;50(3):169–78.

15. Kalemaj Z, Levrini L. Quantitative evaluation of implemented interproximal enamel reduction during aligner therapy. Angle Orthod. 2021;91(1):61–6.

16. Jarjoura K, Gagnon G, Nieberg L. Caries risk after interproximal enamel reduction. Am J Orthod Dentofacial Orthop. 2006;130(1):26–30.

17. Kailasam V, Rangarajan H, Easwaran HN, Muthu MS. Proximal enamel thickness of the permanent teeth: a systematic review and meta-analysis. Am J Orthod Dentofacial Orthop. 2021;160(6):793–804 e3.

18. Zhou N, Guo J. Efficiency of upper arch expansion with the Invisalign system. Angle Orthod. 2020;90(1):23–30.

19. Lione R, Paoloni V, Bartolommei L, Gazzani F, Meuli S, Pavoni C, et al. Maxillary arch development with Invisalign system. Angle Orthod. 2021;91(4):433–40.

20. Levrini L, Carganico A, Abbate L. Maxillary expansion with clear aligners in the mixed dentition: a preliminary study with Invisalign(R) first system. Eur J Paediatr Dent. 2021;22(2):125–8.

21. Ravera S, Castroflorio T, Garino F, Daher S, Cugliari G, Deregibus A. Maxillary molar distalization with aligners in adult patients: a multicenter retrospective study. Prog Orthod. 2016;17:12.

Clinical Management of Class II Division 1 Cases

7

7.1 Introduction

This chapter focuses on the processes that need to be followed for a successful treatment of a class II division 1 malocclusion.

The following descriptions and terminologies are commonly associated with this type of malocclusion.

Definition: When the mandibular incisor edges lie posterior to the cingulum plateau of the maxillary incisors and the maxillary incisors are straight or proclined [1].

Incidence: 20–30% of malocclusions.

Extraoral features:

- Convex profile

Soft tissue features:

- Competent/incompetent lips
- Normal/deep labio-mental sulcus

Intraoral features:

- Incisor relationship: Class II division 1 incisor relationship with an increased overjet greater than 4 mm
- Canine relationship: The mesial incline of the upper canine is mesial to the distal slope of the lower canine (the maxillary canine occludes more anterior to the mandibular canine and the first premolar)
- Molar relationship: The mesio-buccal cusp of the maxillary first permanent molar occludes anterior to the buccal groove of the mandibular first permanent molar

© The Author(s), under exclusive license to Springer Nature Switzerland AG 2024
S. Abela, *Aligner Systems in Invisible Orthodontics*,
https://doi.org/10.1007/978-3-031-49204-4_7

7.2   Align Technology Grading of Case Difficulty

Align Technology, Inc. method of grading class II malocclusions is identical to grading of any other type of aligner cases. Classification of class II cases are as follows:

Mild/simple class II

– Colour code: green
– Antero-posterior (A-P) correctional movements: less than 4 mm
– Dental extractions: none
– Distalisation: less than 2 mm
– Mesialisation: none

Moderate/intermediate class II

– Colour code: blue
– Antero-posterior correctional movements: less than 4 mm
– Dental extractions: none
– Distalisation: between 2 and 4 mm
– Mesialisation: less than 2 mm

Severe/complex class II

– Colour code: black
– Antero-posterior correctional movements: more than 4 mm
– Dental extractions: yes
– Distalisation: more than 4 mm
– Mesialisation: more than 2 mm

In the mildest form, the case is more predictable with less complex movements involved and less than 2 mm individual tooth movements.

For moderate cases, the predictability is more variable with individual tooth movements of between 2 and 4 mm whilst for more complex cases, the predictability is more uncertain with movements potentially exceeding 4 mm.

The software can make allowances for the anticipations with A-P correction using class II elastics with a "virtual jump".

7.3   Predicting Treatment Outcomes

The predictability of class II cases depends on two major factors: the degree of A-P correction needed and the degree of dentoalveolar compensation present.

It is more predictable if a patient with a class II malocclusion presents with the following:

– At the start of an active phase of growth
– A low degree of dental decompensation
– A positive overbite
– Class I buccal segment relationship
– Class I canine relationship

7.4 Formulating the Treatment Plan

At the prescription stage of the treatment, the treating clinician has two important aspects of the malocclusion to determine:

1. The amount of A-P correction needed
2. The treatment methods of obtaining the desired A-P correction

The clinician has 5 A-P correction options in class II cases with aligners. These are listed in chronological order starting from the ones that provides least A-P correction to the ones that creates the most A-P correction:

– Upper labial or buccal segment IPR or a combination of both
– Buccal segment distalisation
– Class II mechanics with inter arch elastics
– Fixed-functional appliances
– TADS-supported distalising appliances
– Dental extractions
– Surgical correction

7.4.1 Class II Elastics

Class II elastic placement, classically placed between the lower first molars to the upper canine region, is very beneficial to the correction of class II malocclusions.

The placement of this auxiliary can be specified within the doctor's preferences section of the ClinCheck® or applied within the prescription form on submission of the case.

The elastic bands can be designed to engage precision cuts within the invisalign tray or alternatively the tray is designed with a cut-out to enable placement of an additional button. Precision cuts can be ordered in combination with conventional or optimised attachments if there is enough tooth surface area.

If sufficient tooth area is not present to accommodate for both design features, the software defaults to prioritising the optimised attachment over the precision cut. If there is a lack of space but enough to allow an attachment and a precision hook, the software will resort to the latter design by default.

7.4.2 Elastic Band Sizes

The treating doctor would have over time, built a more preferred size and type which in their opinion works best. Their effect is undoubtedly positive on the overall malocclusion and should be incorporated in the aligner treatment when indicated [2].

The forces as calculated and interpreted by the manufacturers is equivalent to the force dissipated by the elastic band when they are stretched by three times their lumen size.

Classical types and sizes are indicated below in chronological order of preference:

- Class II elastics from lower first molars to the upper canines: 3/16 in. (5 mm) producing 2.5 ounces of force which is equivalent to 70 g of force.
- Class II elastics from lower first molars to the upper canines: 3/16 in. (5 mm) producing 3.5 ounces of force which is equivalent to 98 g of force.
- Class II elastics from lower first molars to the upper canines: 3/16 in. (5 mm) producing 4.5 ounces of force which is equivalent to 128 g of force.

Additional elastic bands that can be considered especially if the lower second molars are engaged in contrast to the lower first molars:

- Class II elastics from the lower second molars to the upper canines 1/4 in. (6 mm) medium, 3.5 or 4.5 ounces producing 98 and 128 g of force, respectively.
- Class II elastics from the lower second molar to the upper canines 5/16 in. (8 mm) producing 3.5 or 4.5 ounces producing 98 and 128 g of force, respectively.

The choice between the latter two types of elastics for the engagement of lower second molars depends on the distance between these teeth to the precision hooks in the upper canine region.

7.5 Additional Treatment Considerations

Prior to, during or after clear aligner treatment additional treatment considerations could need to be applied by the clinician. These could include the inclusion of fixed-functional appliances, maxillary first molar de-rotations, passive aligners at the end of the active treatment or in the opposing arch to the one being treated and pontic placement in case of missing or previously extracted teeth.

7.5.1 Fixed-Functional Appliances

One of the most widely used fixed-functional devices is the Carriere® Motion 3D™ appliance. Aligner treatment can't considered as the most efficacious method for all types of tooth movements and all types of malocclusions, and this is certainly valid for correction of class II malocclusions in adults [3]. This has classically been used in conjunction with upper and lower fixed appliances on a non-extraction basis; however, its use with aligners most notably Invisalign® has been popularised amongst clinicians. Conceptualised as a distalisation type of appliance, it allows sagittal correction of the buccal segments prior to starting the clear aligner therapy phase. This phase aims to facilitate the use and increase patients' compliance with the aligners by reducing treatment time and improving efficiency of the overall treatment.

7.5.1.1 Indications for the Use of Carriere® Motion 3D™ Appliance

- Class II division 1 or 2 incisor relationship
- Positive overbite
- Unilateral or bilateral class II canine relationship
- Unilateral or bilateral class II molar relationship
- Growing and adult patients [4]

7.5.1.2 Exclusion Criteria for the Use of Carriere® Motion 3D™ Appliance

- Skeletal discrepancy with a retrognathic mandible
- Full unit class II molar relationship suitable for correction with other types of functional appliances
- Dentition affected by periodontal disease

7.5.1.3 Mode of Action of the Carriere® Motion 3D™ Appliance

Most of the effects of conventional functional appliances are dissipated albeit unequally, between skeletal and dental effects. In the case of Carriere® Motion 3D™ appliance, the extraoral effects are extremely limited whilst the intraoral effects are limited to dentoalveolar changes which include the following:

- In the upper arch, distal canine tipping and molar tipping with spacing distal to upper lateral incisors
- In the lower arch, lower incisor proclination leading to improvements in overjet and overbite dimensions [5]

7.5.1.4 Selection of the Carriere® Motion 3D™ Appliance

The device comes in multiple sizes, spaced in 2 mm increments and in stainless steel or clear to render it more discreet. The initial phase of the selection process starts with measuring the mid-point of the molar and canine on the ipsilateral side. The device is directly bonded to the buccal surface of the first molar and extended to the canine or first premolar on the ipsilateral side. In the lower arch, a fixed lower lingual arch with retention arms extending distally to the second molars or mesially to the first premolars can be chosen. Alternatively, the dentition in the lower arch can be covered with an Essix® type of retainer modified to accommodate the molar tubes on the first or second molars.

The recommended intermaxillary elastics is as follows:

1. ¼ in., with a force delivery of 4.5 ounces (oz) for the first 6 weeks
2. ¼ in., 6.0 oz elastics
3. ¼ in., 9.0 oz elastics
4. Intermaxillary elastic use is continued until full correction of the canine and molar relationships is observed

7.5.1.5 Advantages of Using the Carriere® Motion 3D™ Appliance

The advantages of using a combination approach with the Carriere® Motion 3D™ appliance prior to Invisalign® treatment could be inferred by following a two-step approach for class II malocclusions and include the following:

- The sagittal correction is completed in the initial phase.
- Carriere® Motion 3D™ appliance increases the scope of treatment with an increased range of tooth movement rendered possible.
- Increased efficiency of tooth movement.
- Less reliance on molar distalisation with Invisalign®.
- Decreased overall treatment time.
- Assessment of patient compliance.

7.5.1.6 The Aligner Phase Following the Use of the Carriere® Motion 3D™ Appliance

Following the conclusion of the Carriere® Motion 3D™ appliance phase, the main aim of the aligners is to align and close any interdental spacing that would have resulted from the first phase. The spacing is commonly found distal to the upper lateral incisors. The use of optimised attachments in the planning phase will ensure maximum crown and root movement efficiency during this final phase.

The transition phase between the two appliances could necessitate the need of precision cuts usually on the lower first molars and upper canines for the use of class II intermaxillary elastic bands. Clinicians in such cases should include retention attachments with a horizontal bevel on at least one molar in each quadrant. This is usually placed on the most mesial aspect of the lower first molars to avoid impingement in the button area of the same teeth.

Two important aspects to consider following the use of Carriere® Motion 3D™ appliance is the distal tipping of the canine which is associated with relative extrusion and the vertical extrusion of the first or second molars with the use of the intermaxillary elastics with heavier forces of 6–9 oz. The aligner phase should ensure both adequate alignment of the dentition but also good vertical control. In the case of maxillary second molars, prevention of vertical extrusion will allow a favourable counterclockwise auto-rotation of the mandible which will reinforce the skeletal antero-posterior discrepancy.

7.5.2 Upper First Molar De-rotation

It is observed that in the interim phase between primary and mixed dentition phases, with the eruption of the first molars, the latter are associated with mesio-palatal rotation invariably. This is attributed to the mesial migration of the molars following development and obtaining a good contact point with the in-standing upper second deciduous molars. This pattern involving mesial drifting of the first molar is further worsened with a shortened arch due to crowding with buccal or palatal displacement of teeth within the arch.

It should be customary that the clinician requests de-rotation of the first molars in the maxillary arch in a mesio-buccal direction. This allows space creation of up to 2 mm on each side which could be used to align the teeth within the arch and facilitate the attainment of a class I molar relationship.

This technique can also be applied to the upper second molars. Consideration of vertical attachments to these teeth can be put in place if distalisation is needed at the same time.

7.5.3 Passive Aligners in the Opposing Arch

Additional features to consider is ordering passive aligners in the opposing arch in cases where movement in one arch is being planned. This allows any possibility of relapse and better predictability of the final occlusion.

7.5.4 Pontics

In hypodontia or cases where teeth have been lost due to trauma or carious breakdown, the placement of pontics can be requested in the prescription phase. This is used to disguise the missing teeth and maintain the space for the prosthetic replacement.

References

1. British Standards Institute. Glossary of dental terms (BS 4492). London: BSI; 1983.
2. Lombardo L, Colonna A, Carlucci A, Oliverio T, Siciliani G. Class II subdivision correction with clear aligners using intermaxilary elastics. Prog Orthod. 2018;19(1):32.
3. Patterson BD, Foley PF, Ueno H, Mason SA, Schneider PP, Kim KB. Class II malocclusion correction with Invisalign: is it possible? Am J Orthod Dentofacial Orthop. 2021;159(1):e41–e8.
4. Carriere L. A new class II distalizer. J Clin Orthod. 2004;38(4):224–31.
5. Kim-Berman H, McNamara JA Jr, Lints JP, McMullen C, Franchi L. Treatment effects of the Carriere((R)) motion 3D appliance for the correction of class II malocclusion in adolescents. Angle Orthod. 2019;89(6):839–46.

Clinical Management of Class II Division 2 Cases

8

8.1 Introduction

This chapter focuses on the processes that need to be followed for a successful treatment of class II division 2 malocclusions.

The following descriptions and terminologies are commonly associated with this type of malocclusion.

Definition: When the mandibular incisor edges lie posterior to the cingulum plateau of the maxillary incisors with retroclined maxillary incisors or a combination of retroclined maxillary central incisors and proclined lateral incisors [1].

Incidence: 15–20% of malocclusions [2].

Extraoral features:

- Straight profile/convex

Soft tissue features:

- Competent lips
- Normal/deep labio-mental sulcus

Intraoral features:

- Incisor relationship: Class II division 2 incisor relationship. Retroclination of the upper labial segment can affect all incisors or can affect the central incisors only with the upper lateral incisors being proclined. Two further subdivisions of this malocclusion can be identified:

  - Subdivision II division 2(a) with retroclination of all incisors or the central incisors only with a reduced overjet
  - Subdivision II division 2(b) with retroclination of all incisors or the central incisors only with an increased overjet

S. Abela, *Aligner Systems in Invisible Orthodontics*,
https://doi.org/10.1007/978-3-031-49204-4_8

 – Canine relationship: The mesial incline of the upper canine overlaps the distal slope of the lower canine (the maxillary canine occludes between the mandibular canine and the first premolar).
 – Molar relationship: The mesio-buccal cusp of the maxillary first permanent molar occludes in the anterior-buccal groove of the mandibular first permanent molar.

8.2 Align Technology Grading of Case Difficulty

The grading of difficulty based on the amount of tooth movement needed is based on three types of movements: anterior segment intrusion, posterior segment extrusion and whether surgical treatment is needed.

In case anterior intrusion only suffices and the movement is less than 2.5 mm, the case would be considered as simple. In case that posterior extrusion is needed of less than 1 mm in conjunction with anterior intrusion of less than 3 mm, the case is considered as of intermediate difficulty, whilst if the case entails, anterior intrusion and posterior extrusion of more than 3 mm and 1 mm, respectively, the case is considered as a surgical case. This classification is colour-coded as green, blue and black in chronological order of difficulty. This is tabulated below in Table 8.1 below.

8.3 General Concepts

The first consideration when treating class II division 2 cases is the alignment of incisors. The upper labial segment, namely the central and lateral incisors are retroclined in part or in full, that is the upper right and left central and lateral incisors.

The three main stages in obtaining full correction and alignment of the incisors is as follows:

1. Upper incisor (central and/or lateral incisors) proclination
2. Intrusion of the upper incisors—this can be relative or pure intrusion
3. Retraction of the upper labial segment following uprighting due to the alignment and a consequential increase in overjet

The treatment planning in class II division 2 cases revolves primarily around the management of the deep bite. Following the three stages mentioned above, other considerations that need to be undertaken are related to the buccal segments:

Table 8.1 Align Technology, Inc. (San Jose, CA, USA) grading of complexity of a class II case based on the amount of tooth movement needed

Grading of case difficulty	Colour code	Posterior extrusion	Anterior intrusion
1. Simple	Green	No	Less than 2.5 mm
2. Intermediate	Blue	Less than 1 mm	Between 2.5 and 3 mm
3. Complex	Black	More than 1 mm	More than 3 mm

extrusion of the premolar and molars. The levelling of the curve of Spee constitutes this type of movement in isolation or in conjunction with anterior segment intrusion.

8.3.1   Relative Intrusion

With class II division 2 cases, as mentioned earlier in this chapter, retroclination would be visible on the central incisors with or without the inclusion of the lateral incisors. The correction of the angulation following alignment by uprighting the involved incisors will consequentially tip the crowns buccally. This latter movement gives the visual impression that the incisors have intruded with a reduction in the overbite. This is referred to as relative intrusion as it is consequential to the tipping movement.

8.3.2   Pure Intrusion

Pure intrusion can be considered as an antagonistic movement to relative intrusion as it represents bodily intrusion of the affected incisors. This movement obtains factual vertical reduction in the overbite and not only a visual one.

The treatment planning and consideration of the pre-treatment position of the incisors will enable the clinician to assess the best possible movements for the case being considered for clear aligner treatment.

8.4   Features and ClinCheck® Pro 6 Considerations for Deep Bite Correction

Certain features available to the clinician on the ClinCheck® have to be considered to increase the efficiency in managing class II division cases. The sections below describe these features and the optimal way of setting the ClinCheck® during the prescription stage.

8.4.1   Optimised Attachments

The attachments used in class II division 2 cases can be any of the ones listed below in singularity or in congruity.

- Optimised attachments
- Optimised intrusion attachments for incisors (threshold >1 mm)
- Optimised extrusion attachments for premolars (threshold >0.5 mm)
- Extrusion attachments for molars (threshold >0.5 mm)
- Optimised multi-plane attachments (threshold rotation >5°)

8.4.2 Bite Ramps

Align Technology, Inc. Bite Ramps also referred to as Precision Bite Ramps are equivalent to bite turbos used in fixed appliance therapy. Bite turbos' use as an adjunct in orthodontic treatment has become well established over time [3].

Bite turbos can be placed anteriorly or posteriorly. In the former's case their placement can be on the palatal aspect of the upper incisors, more specifically in the cingulum plateau region or on the incisal third of the buccal surfaces of lower incisors. In the latter's case, their placement is on the intersection between the buccal cusps also known as supporting cusps and the nearest occlusal surface of the first molars.

Indications for anterior bite turbos include the following:

- Increased curve of Spee [4]
- Reverse overjet with lower incisor overlaps over the maxillary incisors with or without forward displacement [5]

Indications for posterior bite turbos include the following:

- Anterior open bite [6]
- Unilateral or bilateral posterior crossbites [6]

Their mode of action includes the following:

- Disocclusion of the anterior and posterior teeth for improved efficiency in tooth movement
- Intrusion of lower incisors
- Posterior segment extrusion in the lower arch [7]

The main contraindication is their use in the patients with increased lower third facial height. Their use with the concomitant posterior segment extrusion can lead to less desirable results.

8.4.3 Setting Up the ClinCheck®

During the prescription stage, the clinician needs to indicate the preferences for managing deep bite cases. The following steps will give a clear-cut strategy of how to choose the preferred options.

8.4.3.1 Indicate Areas of Intrusion; Upper and/or Lower Incisors

Selection of intrusion of the incisors will by default trigger placement of optimised attachments on the premolars to avoid dislodgment of the aligners. An intrusive force anteriorly will stimulate an equal and opposite force which would be upwards on the buccal segments.

8.4.3.2 Over Treat Intrusion of Incisors

The intrusion of incisors is a movement that is not replicable on a 1 to 1 ratio from the ClinCheck® simulation to live situation. Over treatment is a widespread recommendation to obtain as close a result as possible to the one suggested by the simulation. Instructions for this overcorrection can vary between prescribing an arbitrary 2 mm overcorrection or specifically requesting a reduced overbite with an overlap of 0.5 mm in the upper central incisor region and an edge-to-edge relationship of the upper lateral incisors to the lower counterparts.

8.4.3.3 Addition of Precision Bite Ramps

The addition of Bite Ramps will preclude the placement of pressure areas along the long axis of the incisors. The software's algorithms override and places Bite Ramps higher in the chronological order of preference to pressure areas. The Bite Ramps are known to exert more pressure by using the occlusal forces of the lower incisors in addition to the forces exerted by the aligners.

8.4.3.4 Over Torque Incisors

Torque similar to intrusion of incisors is another type of tooth movement that clear aligners might not replicate fully and the real live results might vary from those suggested by the simulation. Under torqued upper incisors is a common occurrence with class II division 2 incisors where retroclination of all the incisors or the central incisors is a characteristic feature. Failure to fully torque the incisors may lead to an elongated incisal guidance pathway during protrusion and less than ideal dynamic occlusion. It is widely accepted to prescribe at least 10° of extra torque to prevent under-expression of torque.

8.4.3.5 Application of Class II Intermaxillary Elastics

The effects of intermaxillary elastics in fixed appliances and clear aligners differ due to the different nature of the two types of appliances.

In case of fixed appliances, class II intermaxillary elastics are associated with a few negative side effects. Primarily these include:

- Extrusion of the buccal segments
- Excessive proclination of the lower incisors
- Loss of torque of the upper incisors due the posterior vector exerted by the direction of the elastics

In case of clear aligners, these negative effects are negated by the presence of the aligners themselves with coverage of the occlusal surfaces and in-built prescription.

The use of intermaxillary elastics is encouraged as it will assist the aligners in the antero-posterior correction.

8.4.4   Retainers Post Deep Bite Correction

Two very important design features to consider during the retention phase of a class II division 2 case with a deep bite are the following:

8.4.4.1 Inclusion of Incisor over Intrusion
The prescription submitted to Vivera® retainers can include an overcorrection degree to prevent relapse of the deep bite which usually starts with loss of the improved interincisal angle.

8.4.4.2 Inclusion of Precision Bite Ramps
The use of Precision Bite Ramps during treatment might be suggestive of the need to include this feature in the Vivera® retainers or in the readers' removable retainers of choice.

8.5   Analysing Evidence on the Efficacy of Deep Bite Correction Using Clear Aligner Therapy

Although the available scientific evidence analysing the efficacy of aligners in general is much less available than with fixed appliances, this is even more applicable to deep bite management using this technique.

A previously conducted study using Invisalign® looked specifically at the efficacy of deep bite management using virtual Bite Ramps in adults and compared the outcomes to patients that received fixed appliance therapy. Their findings although pre- and post-treatment changes were positive for both groups, the fixed appliance group experienced a more significant change in the alignment of the curve of Spee [2]. Positive findings were also found in another study with a favourable change in the maxillary mandibular planes angle of 5° suggesting an improvement in the overbite which was reflection in one of the skeletal parameters used to check this [8].

In the same study, a comparison of maxillary incisor intrusion between patients receiving Invisalign® was 0.88 mm in comparison to 1.14 mm in patients that received fixed appliance therapy [2]. In the case of mandibular incisors, the aligner group had incisor intrusion of 2.06 mm in comparison to the fixed appliances group that experienced 1.30 mm intrusion suggesting that Invisalign® could be superior at incisor intrusion.

A different study altogether using cone beam computed tomography to measure the actual true incisor intrusion measured the true efficacy of incisor intrusion at 51.19% whilst the amount of measured correction was 48.81% [9]. This equates to roughly half the amount of projected incisor intrusion with the greatest precision being achieved by maxillary lateral incisors at 58.12% and the lowest precision achieved on mandibular incisors at 44.71%. The authors also concluded that the mean summation of true intrusion was measured at 0.90 mm. This is very much in line with past scientific reports with mean maxillary incisor intrusion of 1.46 and

1.90 mm for mandibular incisors whilst posteriorly this is even more limited with an estimated mean of 0.96 mm [10, 11].

The bite ramps' efficacy in managing deep bites has been highlighted and proven to be a valid feature to obtain lower incisor intrusion [12].

References

1. British Standards Institute. Glossary of dental terms (BS 4492). London: BSI; 1983.
2. Henick D, Dayan W, Dunford R, Warunek S, Al-Jewair T. Effects of Invisalign (G5) with virtual bite ramps for skeletal deep overbite malocclusion correction in adults. Angle Orthod. 2021;91(2):164–70.
3. Alsheikho HO, Jomah D. A simple technique to fabricate bite turbos. J Indian Orthod Soc. 2021;55(3):331–5.
4. Vibhute PJ, Srivastava S, Hazarey PV. Temporary bite-raising crowns. J Clin Orthod. 2006;40(4):224–30. quiz 31
5. Roy AS, Singh GK, Tandon P, De N. An interim bite raiser. Int J Orthod Milwaukee. 2013;24(2):63–4.
6. Kravitz ND, Jorgensen G, Frey S, Cope J. Resin bite turbos. J Clin Orthod. 2018;52(9):456–61.
7. Al-Zoubi EM, Al-Nimri KS. A comparative study between the effect of reverse curve of Spee archwires and anterior bite turbos in the treatment of deep overbite cases. Angle Orthod. 2022;92(1):36–44.
8. Khosravi R, Cohanim B, Hujoel P, Daher S, Neal M, Liu W, et al. Management of overbite with the Invisalign appliance. Am J Orthod Dentofacial Orthop. 2017;151(4):691–9 e2.
9. Al-Balaa M, Li H, Ma Mohamed A, Xia L, Liu W, Chen Y, et al. Predicted and actual outcome of anterior intrusion with Invisalign assessed with cone-beam computed tomography. Am J Orthod Dentofacial Orthop. 2021;159(3):e275–e80.
10. Ng J, Major PW, Heo G, Flores-Mir C. True incisor intrusion attained during orthodontic treatment: a systematic review and meta-analysis. Am J Orthod Dentofacial Orthop. 2005;128(2):212–9.
11. Ng J, Major PW, Flores-Mir C. True molar intrusion attained during orthodontic treatment: a systematic review. Am J Orthod Dentofacial Orthop. 2006;130(6):709–14.
12. Greco M, Rombola A. Precision bite ramps and aligners: an elective choice for deep bite treatment. J Orthod. 2022;49(2):213–20.

Clinical Management of Class III Cases

9

9.1 Introduction

The full potential of the Invisalign® system and its accompanying software can be exploited by the clinician if an extensive knowledge of its features is at hand when treating class III type of malocclusions. Familiarisation with each individual step and methodological use of the software stages ensures a more realistic outcome in line with the digital projection.

This chapter focuses on the processes that need to be followed for a successful treatment of a class III malocclusion.

The following descriptions and terminologies are commonly associated with this type of malocclusion.

Definition: When the mandibular incisor edges lie anterior to the cingulum plateau of the maxillary incisors [1].

Incidence: 5–10% of all malocclusions.

Extraoral features:

- Straight/concave profile

Soft tissue features:

- Competent/incompetent lips
- Normal/flat labio-mental sulcus

Intraoral features:

- Incisor relationship: Class III
- Canine relationship: The mesial incline of the upper canine is distal to the distal slope of the lower canine (the maxillary canine occludes more posterior to the mandibular canine and the first premolar)

© The Author(s), under exclusive license to Springer Nature Switzerland AG 2024
S. Abela, *Aligner Systems in Invisible Orthodontics*,
https://doi.org/10.1007/978-3-031-49204-4_9

– Molar relationship: The mesio-buccal groove of the mandibular first permanent molar lies anterior to the mesio-buccal cusp of the maxillary first permanent molar

9.2   Align Technology Grading of Case Difficulty

Align Technology, Inc. method of grading class III malocclusions is identical to grading of any other type of aligner case. Classification of class III cases are as follows:

Mild/simple class III

– Colour code: green
– Antero-posterior (A-P) correctional movements: less than 4 mm
– Dental extractions: none
– Distalisation: less than 2 mm
– Mesialisation: none

Moderate/intermediate class III

– Colour code: blue
– Antero-posterior correctional movements: less than 4 mm
– Dental extractions: none
– Distalisation: between 2 and 4 mm
– Mesialisation: less than 2 mm

Severe/complex class III

– Colour code: black
– Antero-posterior correctional movements: more than 4 mm
– Dental extractions: yes
– Distalisation: more than 4 mm
– Mesialisation: more than 2 mm

Table 9.1 below tabulates the complexity levels based on the amount of tooth movement required as classified by Align Technology (San Jose, CA, USA).

Table 9.1 Align Technology, Inc. (San Jose, CA, USA) grading the complexity of a class III case based on the amount of tooth movement needed

Grading of case difficulty	Colour code	Antero-posterior correction	Premolar extraction	Distalisation	Mesialisation
1. Simple	Green	Less than 4 mm	No	Less than 2 mm	No
2. Intermediate	Blue	Less than 4 mm	No	Between 2 and 4 mm	Less than 2 mm
3. Complex	Black	More than 4 mm	Yes	More than 4 mm	More than 2 mm

In the mildest form, the case is more predictable with less complex movements involved and less than 2 mm individual tooth movements.

For moderate cases, the predictability is more variable with individual tooth movements of between 2 and 4 mm whilst for more complex cases, the predictability is more uncertain with movements potentially exceeding 4 mm.

Further difficulty is associated with the presence of a displacement and the clinician needs to identify this from the start and specify it in the ClinCheck®. Features such as initial contact and degree of displacement need to be specified.

The software can make allowances for the anticipations with the correction of the displacement with a "virtual jump".

9.3   Predicting Treatment Outcomes

The predictability of class III cases depend on two major factors: the patient's phase of active growth and the degree of dentoalveolar compensation present.

It is more predictable if a patient with a class III malocclusion presents with the following:

- At the end or complete active phase of growth
- A low degree of dental decompensation
- A positive overbite
- Class I buccal segment relationship
- Presence of a forward contact point displacement into ICP

9.4   Formulating the Treatment Plan

At the prescription stage of the treatment, the treating clinician has two important aspects of the malocclusion to determine:

1. The amount of A-P correction needed
2. The treatment methods of obtaining the desired A-P correction

The clinician has 5 A-P correction options in class III cases with aligners. These are listed in chronological order starting from the ones that provides least A-P correction to the ones that creates the most A-P correction:

- Lower labial segment IPR, buccal segment IPR or a combination of both
- Buccal segment distalisation
- Class III mechanics
- Fixed-functional appliances
- TADS-supported distalising appliances
- Dental extractions
- Surgical correction

Additional features to consider is to order passive aligners in the opposing arch in cases where movement in one arch is being planned.

Reference

1. British Standards Institute. Glossary of dental terms (BS 4492). London: BSI; 1983.

Clinical Management of Anterior Open Bite Cases   10

10.1   Introduction

The presence of an anterior open bite is very frequently obvious to both the clinician and the patient alike. It also very frequently affects both the smile aesthetics and the function equally. The diagnosis of the aetiological factor or factors is key to managing these types of cases.

The following descriptions and terminologies are commonly associated with this type of malocclusion.

Prevalence rate in adolescents: 16.52% [1].

Extraoral features:

– Straight/convex profile

Soft tissue features:

– Incompetent lips
– Normal/deep labio-mental sulcus

Intraoral features:

– Incisor relationship: Predominantly class I or class II division 1 cases although can also present in class III cases
– Symmetrical open bites
– Asymmetrical open bites: Digit sucking habit (present/past)

10.2   Align Technology Grading of Case Difficulty

Align Technology, Inc. (San Jose, CA, USA) method of grading class III malocclusions is identical to grading of any other type of aligner case. Classification of class III cases are as follows:

Mild/simple anterior open bite

- Colour code: green
- Anterior extrusion: less than 2.5 mm
- Dental extractions: none
- Posterior intrusion: none
- Surgery: not indicated

Moderate/intermediate anterior open bite

- Colour code: blue
- Anterior extrusion: less than 2.5 mm
- Dental extractions: none
- Posterior intrusion: less than 1 mm
- Surgery: not indicated

Severe/complex anterior open bite

- Colour code: black
- Anterior extrusion: less than 2.5 mm
- Dental extractions: yes
- Posterior intrusion: more than 1 mm
- Surgery: a viable treatment option

Table 10.1 tabulates the degree of complexity based on the amount of tooth movement required.

In the mildest form, the case is more predictable with less complex movements involving less than 2.5 mm of anterior extrusion with no posterior intrusion and no indications for surgical treatment.

For moderate cases, the predictability is more variable with incisor extrusive movements of less than 2.5 mm and posterior intrusion of less than 1 mm. For more complex cases, the predictability is more uncertain with extrusive movements

Table 10.1 Align Technology, Inc. (San Jose, CA, USA) grading of complexity of an open bite case based on the amount of tooth movement needed

Grading of case difficulty	Colour code	Surgery	Posterior intrusion	Anterior extrusion
1. Simple	Green	No	No	Less than 2.5 mm
2. Intermediate	Blue	No	Less than 1 mm	Less than 2.5 mm
3. Complex	Black	Yes	More than 1 mm	More than 2.5 mm

anteriorly of more than 2 mm, posterior intrusion of more than 1 mm and surgical treatment could be justified.

Further difficulty is associated with the presence of the following:

– A persistent digit sucking habit
– An active growth spurt
– Skeletal discrepancies with increased lower facial height
– An unfavourable growth pattern with a backward growth rotation of the mandible

The software even in anterior open bite cases can make allowances for the anticipations with the correction of the displacement with a "virtual jump".

10.3 Predicting Treatment Outcomes

Following from the section above listing the features that could render a case more complex, the predictability of anterior open bite cases primarily depends on three major factors: the patient's phase of active growth, the pattern of skeletal growth and the degree of dentoalveolar compensation present.

It is more predictable if a patient with an anterior open bite malocclusion presents with the following:

– No active habits and/or habits stopped in the primary dentition stage
– No visible tongue thrust
– At the end or complete active phase of growth
– A high degree of dental decompensation
– Presence of interdental spacing
– Class I buccal segment relationship

10.4 Formulating the Treatment Plan

At the prescription stage of the treatment, the treating clinician has two important treatment planning aspects to consider:

1. The biomechanics needed to address the malocclusion. This is determined by assessing two important factors:
   (a) The amount of vertical and A-P correction needed
   (b) The treatment methods of obtaining the desired vertical and A-P correction if the indicated
2. The aesthetic changes needed for the case by anticipating the final treatment results:
   (a) The amount of incisal and gingival display at rest and on smiling
   (b) The levelling and alignment of the upper incisors and smile aesthetics in relation to the lower lip

10.4.1 Type of Tooth Movements to Manage an Anterior Open Bite

The tooth movements for an anterior open bite correction could be classified into three broad categories:

- Relative incisor extrusion
- Pure incisor extrusion
- Intrusion of the posterior segments

10.4.1.1 Relative Incisor Extrusion

Relative incisor extrusion is accomplished with retroclination of the upper incisors. This type of movement is indicated in the presence of proclined upper incisors pretreatment, with interdental spacing. In caucasians the presence of an incisor inclination to the maxillary plane greater than 109° ± 6° is a good indication. By tipping the crown of the incisors lingually, relative extrusion is obtained improving the vertical relationship of the labial segments and thus improving the overbite simultaneously.

In case that present with proclined incisors however there is lack of interdental spacing, IPR would need to be prescribed to obtain relative extrusion. Figure 10.1 below illustrates the principle of relative incisor extrusion.

10.4.1.2 Pure Incisor Extrusion

Pure incisor extrusion refers to the bodily movement of the upper and/or lower incisors in a vertical plane. This movement is indicated when the upper incisors to the maxillary plane and the lower incisors to the mandibular plane are of average inclinations; 109° ± 6° and 90° ± 5°, respectively. Figure 10.2 below illustrates the principle of pure incisor extrusion.

Fig. 10.1 Relative incisor extrusion

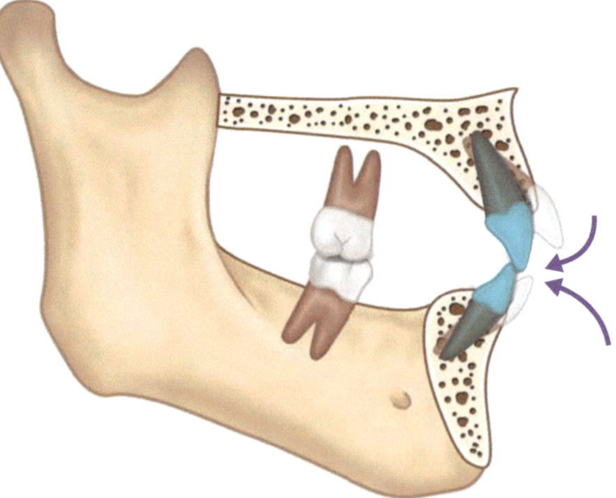

Fig. 10.2 Pure incisor
extrusion

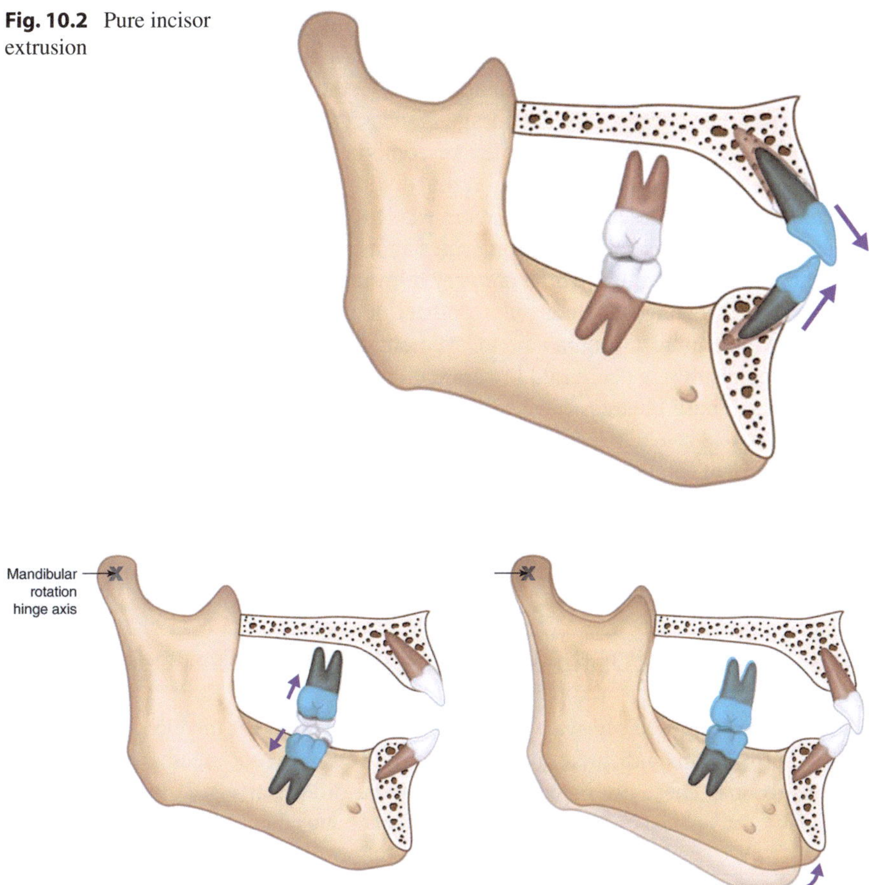

Fig. 10.3 Molar intrusion causing anticlockwise rotation of the mandible

10.4.1.3   Intrusion of the Posterior Segments

Intrusion of posterior segments refers to intrusion of molars unless there is an occlusal step involving all the teeth in the buccal segment including the premolar segment. Intrusion of the posterior teeth allows an alteration of the occlusal plane with a favourable counterbalancing movement of the incisors and an anticlockwise autorotation of the mandible which assists further in improving the overbite. It has been estimated that the ratio of reciprocal anterior open bite closure to molar intrusion is as high as three to one [2]. Similar conclusions and measurements of 2.6 mm were obtained in a separate study carried out by Kim et al. 2018 [3]. Figure 10.3 below illustrates the anticlockwise rotation of the mandible following molar intrusive movements.

10.4.1.4 Anticlockwise Auto-rotation of the Mandible

The intrusion of posterior segments described above will inevitably lead to an anticlockwise auto-rotation of the mandible [4]. Orthodontic mini-implants (OMIs) also referred to as temporary anchorage devices (TADS) have rendered this treatment modality more successful often in combination to fixed appliance therapy. OMIs have also been successfully combined with clear aligners and have obtained very good success rates [5]. This anticlockwise rotation of the mandible also referred to as counterclockwise auto-rotation brings about changes in principally three skeletal and one dental feature which are very relevant to closure of AOBs.

The skeletal changes include antero-posterior changes with a more forward positioning of the chin resulting in an improvement in a class II skeletal base. The vertical changes result in a decreased lower facial height and thus a decrease in overbite dimensions. These changes have to be factored in as molar intrusion in a patient with a class III skeletal base would result in an unfavourable A-P change.

The centre of rotation of the mandible with molar intrusion lies behind and below Condylion (Co), the most lateral point on the surface of the condyle. This was also measured scientifically by the same team mentioned above at 7.4 mm behind and 16.9 mm below Co [3].

10.5 Treatment Options for Managing an Anterior Open Bite

The clinician can be faced with several treatment options for the closure of AOBs. If A-P correction is indicated, most commonly AOBs present together with class II malocclusions. These are listed in chronological order starting from the ones that provides least vertical correction to the ones that creates the most vertical correction:

- Lower and/or upper labial segment IPR, buccal segment IPR or a combination of both
- Lingual crown tipping during interdental space closure
- Buccal segment distalisation
- Class III mechanics
- TADS-supported molar intrusion mechanics/devices
- Dental extractions
- Surgical correction

10.6 Unwanted Molar Intrusion with Aligners

This section specifically describes the commonly visualised effect of clear aligner treatment, unwanted molar intrusion. This is witnessed in most cases treated.

10.6.1 Treatment-Induced Molar Intrusion with Aligners

A degree of unwanted or unplanned molar intrusion is often the norm with clear aligner therapy. This is mainly attributable to the thickness of the aligners which in the case of Invisalign® by Align Technology, Inc. (Santa Clara, CA, USA) each tray is 0.75 mm in thickness, rendering the total inter arch disocclusion by 1.5 mm. The requested wear time of 22 h each day is also a contributory factor. In a retrospective study specifically analysing the molar intrusion with Invisalign® aligners has shown that three quarters of the patients experienced this or 74.2% to be very precise with the intrusion being located in the maxilla, in the mandible or both [6]. The amount of intrusion affecting the upper molars was 0.98 mm with a standard deviation of 0.54 mm, whereas the amount of intrusion affecting the mandibular molars was 0.84 mm with a deviation of 0.29 mm. The measurements obtained in a different study indicated a mean maxillary molar intrusion of 0.4 mm and a mean mandibular intrusion of 0.6 mm [2].

10.6.2 Management of Unwanted Molar Intrusion with Aligners

Additional active treatment following completion of the planned aligner course is not usually indicated to correct the molar intrusion associated with treatment. This is ideally managed conservatively in either of the ways listed below:

- Trimming the upper and/or lower active trays in the buccal segments; The final tray can be trimmed in the premolar region to allow buccal segment settling.
- Decrease the amount of tray wear each day to half; Once the active treatment is completed the patient can be instructed to decrease the amount of wear to at least half the recommended amount, 10–12 h.
- Use the last tray as a retainer until buccal segment settling is complete; The last tray in the treatment batch can be used as a retainer and worn at nighttime only to retain the position of the teeth.
- Provide retainers which allow better buccal settling. These can be Hawley Retainers [7] or Begg Retainers [8]. These are illustrated in Fig. 10.4 below.
- Modify Vacuum-Formed Retainers (VFRs) to allow occlusal hollowing; Vacuum-formed retainers can be modified by hollowing the occlusal surfaces within the buccal segments [9]. This has been shown to improve the inter arch occlusal contact; however, they are rendered weaker with a greater risk of fracture of the retainers [10]. These are illustrated in Fig. 10.5 below.
- Provide Fixed/Bonded retainers; Bonded retainers have been shown to allow even greater buccal segment settling than Hawley retainers [11].

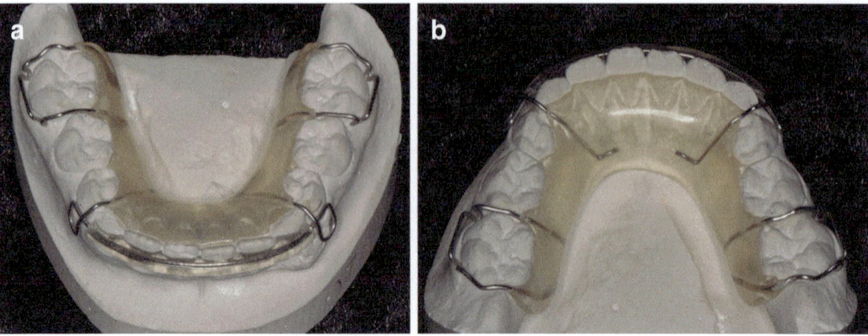

Fig. 10.4 (**a**) Anterior view of a Lower Hawley Retainer with an acrylate labial bow. (**b**) Posterior view of a Lower Hawley Retainer with an acrylate labial bow. (This figure has been reproduced by kind permission of the author, Dr. Stefan Abela)

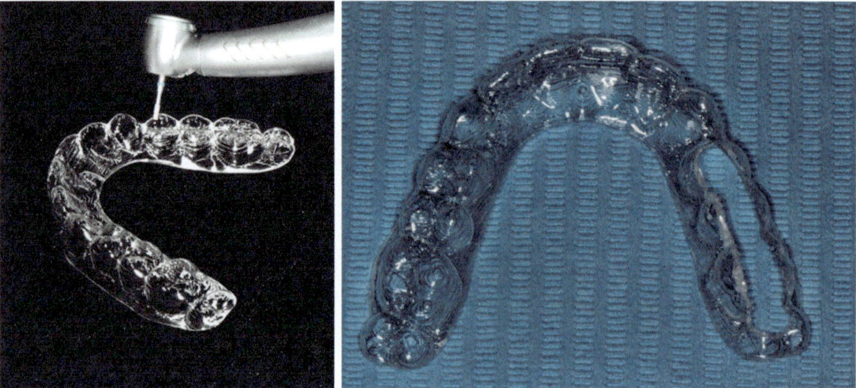

Fig. 10.5 Modified vacuum-formed retainers (VFRs) by eliminating the occlusal coverage of the retainer from the posterior segment. This can be done chair-side or submitted in the prescription to the supplier. The modification can be applied to the upper VFR only or to both upper and lower VFRs. (This figure has been reproduced by kind permission of the author, Dr. Stefan Abela)

10.6.3 Positive Aspects of Unwanted Molar Intrusion with Aligners

The advantage of this iatrogenic aspect of clear aligner treatment is threefold:

1. Active treatment is rarely indicated.
2. Intermolar clearance at the end of the active treatment can favourably support relapse without a detrimental effect on the vertical overlap of the incisors.
3. Patients do not report discomfort or functional compromise with a lack of contact between the molars.

10.7   Features and ClinCheck® Pro 6 Considerations for Anterior Open Bite Correction

10.7.1   Optimised Attachments

Optimised attachments for AOB closure can be:

1. Singular—Placed on single anterior teeth, indicated for asymmetric open bites involving individual teeth. The threshold for inclusion by the software's algorithm is 0.5 mm and is available for both incisors and canines. Figure 10.6a illustrates this below.
2. Multiple—Placed on multiple or all the incisors to obtain extrusion of the labial segment. The threshold for inclusion is also 0.5 mm however is only available for the upper and lower incisors. Figure 10.6b illustrates this below.

10.7.2   Positioning of Attachments

The placement of optimised attachments should be placed adjacent to teeth that need intrusion. This tactical placement of the attachments will ensure that vertical anchorage is provided close to the active site of intrusion and will also provide additional retention to the trays.

10.7.3   Incomplete Levelling of the Arches

Very similarly to fixed appliances' biomechanics when a case presents with an AOB, residual positive curves of Spee in both arches are favourable. This is usually introduced by inserting positively curved round stainless steel archwires to increase the overbite. In surgical cases, this is accomplished by positively curving a rectangular stainless steel.

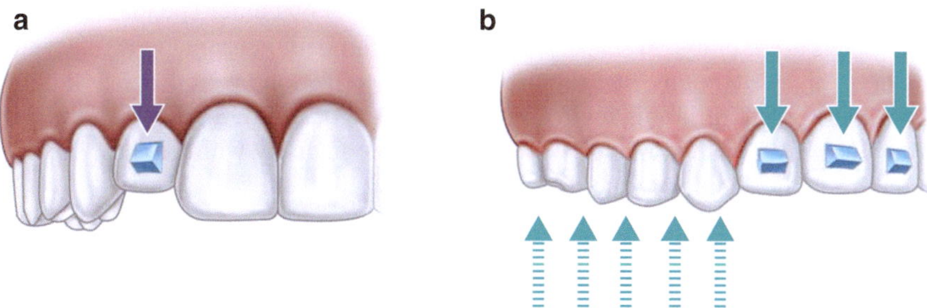

Fig. 10.6 (**a**) Single optimised attachment. (**b**) Multiple optimised attachments

In clear aligner therapy, the concept is identical with positively curves of Spee accepted rather than full levelling to keep an increased overlap of the incisors for full correction and in anticipation of a degree of relapse. Further details about relapse in AOB cases can be found below in Sect. 10.8.

10.7.4 Maxillary Expansion

Cases presenting with AOBs on a class II skeletal base and with increased overjet would benefit from maxillary expansion in the premolar and molar segments. Buccal segment expansion will not only address the transverse component but the A-P component as well.

- Transverse component: Uprighting palatally tipped posterior teeth would correct any posterior cross bite and will also allow an optimal final occlusion and periodontal health. Caution is needed not to over expand the buccal segments as this could lead to extrusion of the palatal cusps and cause occlusal interferences with the buccal cusps on the mandibular molars.
- A-P component: Maxillary expansion of the buccal segments will provide a broader arch increasing the overall arch perimeter with a concomitant arch length reduction. This increase in arch perimeter with a resultant arch length reduction will consequentially decrease the labial segment protrusion by allowing upper incisors lingual crown tipping. This palatal movement of the upper incisors was described very well by a study specifically analysing the effects of maxillary expansion on the arch perimeter [12]. The impact of upper arch expansion labially was measured at 0.4 mm ± 5 mm which was in line with other studies [13].

10.7.5 Monitoring Tracking Closely

Although monitoring of any loss of aligner tracking is crucial at every stage of treatment, in AOB cases, this could be considered even more so. Any loss of tracking or ill-fitting of the tray over the molars could lead to a reduction in the intended magnitude of intrusion which will lead to an unsuccessful outcome. The maxillary second molars are rhombic in shape and usually smaller in dimension to maxillary first molars. This is a common site for an aligner to lose tracking with the patient noticing a less precise fit in this region, unilaterally or bilaterally. This is also the case when the maxillary first molars were extracted prematurely with maxillary second and third molars being present in the molar region.

10.7.6 A-P and Vertical Anchorage Considerations During AOB Closure

In case of missing maxillary first molars, the A-P and vertical anchorage provided by second and third molars will be less than that provided by the maxillary first molars. The reason for this is twofold:

- The maxillary second molars have a reduced dimensional aspect in comparison to maxillary first molars. The impact of size is even greater in third molars with the crown morphology being more rhomboid and smaller in both occluso-cervically and mesio-distally.
- The roots are less divergent in maxillary second molars and frequently fused. Third molars exhibit an even greater frequency of radicular fusion and thus provide the least anchorage reinforcement.

10.8 Relapse Rates of Anterior Open Bites

A well-known sequel of anterior open bite treatment is relapse; this can be minimal or significant enough for patients to seek additional courses of treatment. Several factors can play a part in this propensity for relapse, following successful treatment. Skeletally, increased lower facial heights, persistent digit sucking habits or tongue posture are considered high risk factors [14]. This is equally valid for both surgical and non-surgically corrected cases. Past figures reported that relapse was seen albeit to varying degrees in roughly one third of treated cases [15]. More contemporaneous studies observe relapse in around one quarter of treated cases [16]. These figures are important so the information can be relayed to the patient and an informed consent obtained to having treatment or declining it.

10.9 Retainer Considerations for Maintenance of Anterior Open Bite Closure

The notoriety of relapse in anterior open bite cases has been investigated numerous times, with the aim of establishing factors that increase the susceptibility of a case relapsing to any degree. Fixed retainers do not suffice in maintaining stability further measures are ideally taken at the end of active treatment [17].

Variations in the treatment therapy such as extraction and non-extraction approaches in fixed appliance therapy did not show significant differences in relapse rates although extraction approaches proved to demonstrate superior stability [18].

Past approaches include the use of high pull headgears, modified functional appliances, and removable appliances with buccal segment occlusal coverage.

In case of suspected abnormal tongue posturing, modified removable appliances with tongue grids have been reportedly beneficial in controlling relapse [19, 20]. Figure 10.7 below illustrates the inclusion of tongue grids.

Suggestions to increase stability include skeletal retention involving the placement of four orthodontic mini-implants in the inter-radicular space of upper and lower lateral incisors and canines [21].

Modifying VFRs to include a posterior bite plan to maintain intrusion of buccal segments has also been suggested. Figure 10.8 below illustrates this technique.

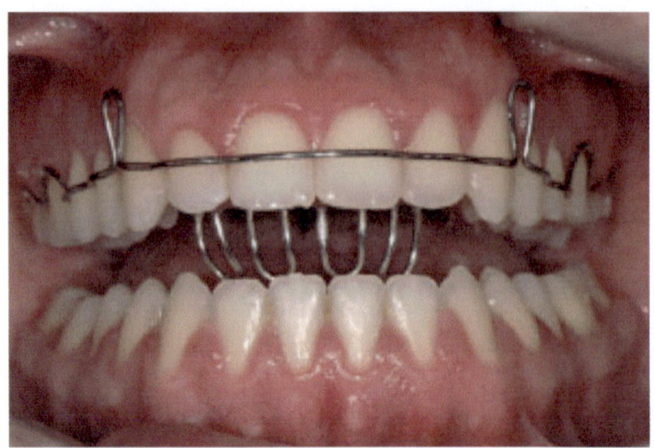

Fig. 10.7 The inclusion of tongue grids in cases of suspected abnormal tongue posturing. (This diagram will reprodcued by kind permission of SAGE)

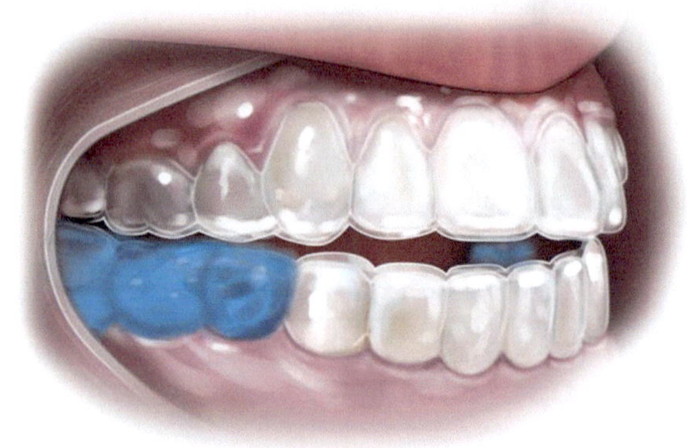

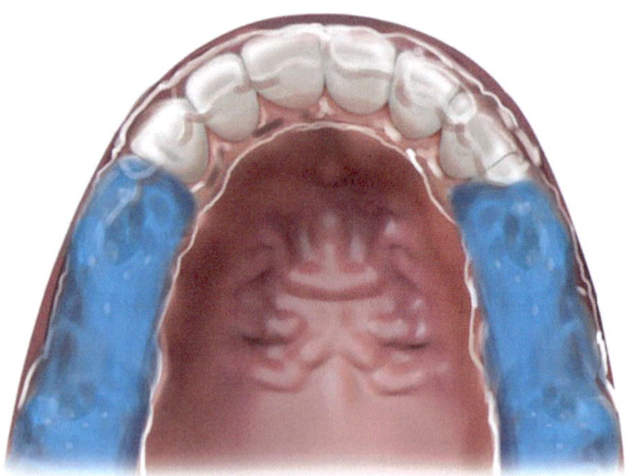

Fig. 10.8 Modification of VFRs with a posterior bite plane to maintain intrusion of molars and premolars. (Figure reproduced by kind permission of Journal of Clinical Orthodontics and courtesy to Dr. Basil Mumtaz)

References

1. Avrella MT, Zimmermann DR, Andriani JSP, Santos PS, Barasuol JC. Prevalence of anterior open bite in children and adolescents: a systematic review and meta-analysis. Eur Arch Paediatr Dent. 2022;23(3):355–64.
2. Moshiri S, Araujo EA, McCray JF, Thiesen G, Kim KB. Cephalometric evaluation of adult anterior open bite non-extraction treatment with Invisalign. Dental Press J Orthod. 2017;22(5):30–8.
3. Kim K, Choy K, Park YC, Han SY, Jung H, Choi YJ. Prediction of mandibular movement and its center of rotation for nonsurgical correction of anterior open bite via maxillary molar intrusion. Angle Orthod. 2018;88(5):538–44.
4. Abuzinada S, Alsulaimani F. Mandibular changes associated with maxillary impaction and molar intrusion. Open J Stomatol. 2013;3:515–9.
5. Park YC, Lee SY, Kim DH, Jee SH. Intrusion of posterior teeth using mini-screw implants. Am J Orthod Dentofacial Orthop. 2003;123(6):690–4.
6. Talens-Cogollos L, Vela-Hernandez A, Peiro-Guijarro MA, Garcia-Sanz V, Montiel-Company JM, Gandia-Franco JL, et al. Unplanned molar intrusion after Invisalign treatment. Am J Orthod Dentofacial Orthop. 2022;162(4):451–8.
7. Destang DL, Kerr WJ. Maxillary retention: is longer better? Eur J Orthod. 2003;25(1):65–9.
8. Littlewood SJ, Mitchell L. An introduction to orthodontics. Oxford university Press; 2019.
9. Pithon MM. A modified thermoplastic retainer. Prog Orthod. 2012;13(2):195–9.
10. Ragunanthanan LMU, Vijayalakshmi D. Comparison of settling of occlusion in modified and full coverage thermoplastic retainers using T-scan. APOS Trends Orthod. 2022;12:115–24.
11. Sari Z, Uysal T, Basciftci FA, Inan O. Occlusal contact changes with removable and bonded retainers in a 1-year retention period. Angle Orthod. 2009;79(5):867–72.
12. Adkins MD, Nanda RS, Currier GF. Arch perimeter changes on rapid palatal expansion. Am J Orthod Dentofacial Orthop. 1990;97(3):194–9.
13. Wertz RA. Skeletal and dental changes accompanying rapid midpalatal suture opening. Am J Orthod. 1970;58(1):41–66.
14. Ng CS, Wong WK, Hagg U. Orthodontic treatment of anterior open bite. Int J Paediatr Dent. 2008;18(2):78–83.
15. Lopez-Gavito G, Wallen TR, Little RM, Joondeph DR. Anterior open-bite malocclusion: a longitudinal 10-year postretention evaluation of orthodontically treated patients. Am J Orthod. 1985;87(3):175–86.
16. Greenlee GM, Huang GJ, Chen SS, Chen J, Koepsell T, Hujoel P. Stability of treatment for anterior open-bite malocclusion: a meta-analysis. Am J Orthod Dentofacial Orthop. 2011;139(2):154–69.
17. Salehi P, Pakshir HR, Hoseini SA. Evaluating the stability of open bite treatments and its predictive factors in the retention phase during permanent dentition. J Dent (Shiraz). 2015;16(1):22–9.
18. Janson G, Valarelli FP, Henriques JF, de Freitas MR, Cancado RH. Stability of anterior open bite nonextraction treatment in the permanent dentition. Am J Orthod Dentofacial Orthop. 2003;124(3):265–76. quiz 340
19. Tanimoto K, Suzuki A, Nakatani Y, Yanagida T, Tanne Y, Tanaka E, et al. A case of anterior open bite with severely narrowed maxillary dental arch and hypertrophic palatine tonsils. J Orthod. 2008;35(1):5–15.
20. Farret MM, Farret MM, Farret AM. Skeletal class III and anterior open bite treatment with different retention protocols: a report of three cases. J Orthod. 2012;39(3):212–23.
21. Albaker BRB, Wong R. A new skeletal retention system for retaining anterior open bites. APOS Trends Orthod. 2013;3:49–53.

Clinical Management of Interceptive and Teenage Cases

11

11.1 Introduction

Conventionally, teenage cases are treated with fixed appliances. In certain cases, where indicated, treatment would start in the early mixed dentition as an interceptive phase of treatment to correct certain aspects of occlusion prior to the definitive course of treatment. In class II cases, the fixed appliance phase would ensue following a separate and complementary phase of functional appliances. This is generally in the form of functional appliances such as modified Clarke Twin Block appliances or by using the Herbst appliance. Invisalign® mandibular advancement treatment replicates the same mechanism as the previously mentioned class II correctors however aims to be more comfortable, more discreet and less reliant on class II elastic use by the patient in the final fixed appliance phase. One advantage of the mandibular advancement appliance from Align Technology, Inc. (San Jose, CA, USA) over fixed appliance counterparts is the reduced risk of breakages and hence the need for less emergency appointments provision. On the other hand, its accuracy and efficacy have been questioned at a clinical level. More details on MA can be found in Sect. 11.5 below.

11.2 Classical Treatments Carried Out in Children and Teenagers with Aligners

Children that present with malocclusions that can be treated by interceptive treatment are classically aged between 6 and 10 and present in an early mixed dentition phase. Treatment at this early stage is aimed at facilitating treatment at a later stage and developing the arches further.

The full list of indications for treatment are as follows:

- Antero-posteriorly:
  - Protrusion of maxillary incisors from teeth from habit.
  - Labial segment crossbites involving the incisors only

S. Abela, *Aligner Systems in Invisible Orthodontics*,
https://doi.org/10.1007/978-3-031-49204-4_11

- Labial segment crossbite with soft tissue dehiscences associated with the lower incisors
- Mild malocclusions with forward displacements on closure
- Vertically:
  - Mild to moderate anterior open bite developed from a habit
- Transversely:
  - Unilateral or bilateral posterior crossbite of the upper first molar with or without involving the deciduous molars
  - Constricted maxillary arch
- Dentoalveolar disproportion:
  - Diastema between the upper central incisors
  - Minor interdental spaces interspersed between permanent incisors
  - Mild degree of crowding
  - Displaced teeth commonly lingually displaced lower incisor

In the case of Invisalign First™, the overall scope for the appliance use is to align the erupted dentition, improve the arch shape, maintain space for the erupting dentition and facilitate the later stages of treatment.

11.3 Advantages and Disadvantages of Offering Early Aligner Treatment

There are several advantages in considering interceptive treatment. This type of treatment can be beneficial if planned in advance for the definitive treatment.

In general, Invisalign First® or other types of aligners offering an early-stage treatment can offer patients a better solution to maintain a good level of oral hygiene during treatment. Comfort, the overall treatment journey, and CAD-CAM technology could also feature as superior to other existing systems.

Below is a list of advantages and disadvantages for considering this two-staged approach.

Advantages:

- Minimise the amount of definitive orthodontic treatment needed
- Address aesthetic concerns from an early stage
- Enable growth modification
- Enable patient acclimatisation to orthodontic treatment
- Provide a smooth transition between the mixed and the permanent dentition stages
- Establish a longer rapport with the patient

Disadvantages:

- Incurred fees
- Patient compliance to wear the aligners and change

- Overall treatment time might not be different to other orthodontic systems
- Need for frequent refinement stages due to exfoliation of multiple deciduous teeth
- Lack of retention or aligner efficiency due to partial eruption or short clinical crowns
- Loss of motivation due to lengthy approach
- More frequent episodes of breakages or loss due to extracurricular activities

11.4 Important Invisalign Features During Early Phases of Treatment

The use of Invisalign Firstn® requires as a minimum, the full eruption of the first permanent molars and at least any two incisors that are at least two-thirds erupted. The patients selected to have this interceptive aligner phase should also have at least two primary teeth or unerupted permanent teeth per quadrant in at least three of the four quadrants.

11.4.1 Eruption Compensation (EC)

Invisalign® provides a ClinCheck® feature, Eruption Compensation (EC) with proprietary eruption compensation algorithms available for upper incisors, canines and premolars. It can be applied to lower incisors however no algorithmic calculation is available. The clinician has to be knowledgeable in the leeway space development and space analysis to predict the excessive space or shortage needed for the establishment of a full secondary dentition.

11.4.2 Terminal Molar Tab

Terminal molar tabs is an aligner feature available with Invisalign® that helps prevent supra-eruption of the terminal molars. The eruption tab commonly applied to partially erupted molars, in most cases being first molars displaying delayed eruption pathways or second molars. It is designed to extend over the mesial cusp of the terminal erupting molar. In the case of second molars, the aligner material helps prevent the occlusal surface of the molar from exceeding the height of the first molar. This is akin to a metal rest in removable retainers which is placed on the mesio-occlusal aspect of second molars to prevent further eruption.

11.4.3 Attachments for Primary Teeth

The attachments used on primary teeth are automatically selected by the algorithms in-built within the ClinCheck® software. These can be placed for interceptive

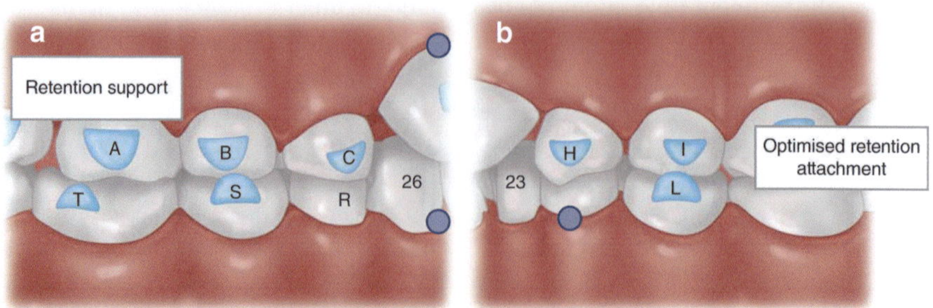

Fig. 11.1 (**a**, **b**) Attachments used on primary teeth for expansion and retention

maxillary expansion in or for tray retention. Figure 11.1a, b demonstrates the two types of attachments below.

11.5 Invisalign Mandibular Advancement (MA)

Description: Invisalign® MA is a type of class II corrector using modified customised trays with precision wings that complement each other between the arches.

Indication: Class II malocclusion with class II division 1 or class II division two subtypes on a class II skeletal base with a retrognathic mandible.

Mode of action: Predominantly dentoalveolar with a very minimal skeletal change estimated to be up to 1° of maxillary arch restraint measured at SNA point and a mandibular growth of up to 1 mm/year.

Threshold: Align Technology, Inc. (Santa Clara, CA, USA) requests that the following clinical criteria are met; at least 2 mm overjet present, less than 7 mm deep bite, more than 3 mm clinical crown height in general and males and/or females that haven't matured skeletally.

Start of MA: The initiation of the MA in the treatment sequence depends on each individual case; however, the initial phase always consists of levelling and aligning and deep bite management before starting the phase with MA.

Classical stages of MA treatment:

- Decompensation of upper incisors in class II division 2 cases and management of deep bite referred to as the pre-MA aligner phase.
- A-P advancement of the mandible with Invisalign® MA to improve the patient's profile and limit the quantity of class II elastics needed during the subsequent stages of treatment.
- Finish arch coordination with additional Aligners.
- Retention—Vivera® retainers and consideration given to incorporating precision bite ramps to maintain a decreased curve of Spee.

Efficacy of MA: The efficacy and accuracy can be questionable with a study reporting a 1.5 mm improvement in overjet reduction over 9 months of wearing MA [1]. This could be considered as clinically not significant and inferior to more conventional class II appliances designed to correct class II malocclusions.

A prospective clinical study has shown that MA works predominantly by affecting the dentoalveolar complex rather than the skeletal elements. Its efficiency has also been proven to be similar to conventional functional appliances [2].

Sagittal correction in teenage patients that present with a class II malocclusion in favour of aligners over conventional fixed appliances are also not disadvantaged. Class II elastic use in teenagers being treated with class II elastics and aligners have been proven to be as efficient as conventional appliances with the added advantage of more control the degree of lower incisor proclination [3]. This advantage has also been reported with the use of MA with better control of lower incisor proclination. On a speculative level, the latter could potentially lessen the dentoalveolar effects and degree of camouflage in favour of skeletal correction [4].

11.6 Retainers in Teenage Cases

Retainers for teenagers might have to be given extra planning due to the continuous changes to the dentition and to cater for the transition between primary and secondary dentition.

One such retainer is the Theroux retainer. Figure 11.2 below illustrates this type of retainer. Its main indication is very early interceptive treatment in 6–8-year-old

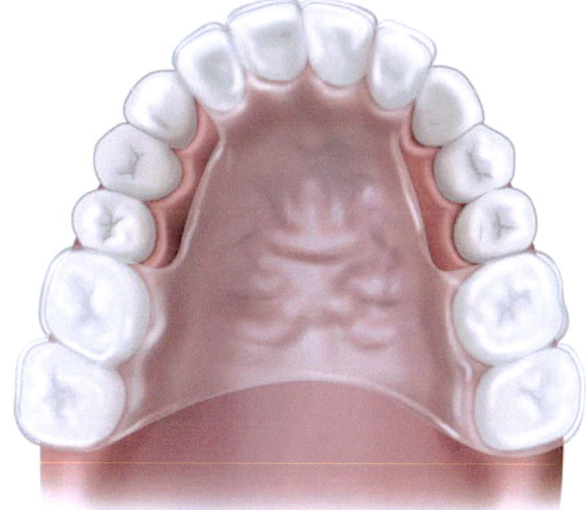

Fig. 11.2 The Theroux retainer. (The image has been kindly replicated from: Removable orthodontic retainers: practical considerations; BDJ, June 11, 2011. Rights reserved by Springer Nature)

patients with the eruption of the permanent incisors and first molars. The indications, design and fabrication methods of this type of retainer are well described in the literature [5].

References

1. Sabouni W, Hansa I, Al Ali SM, Adel SM, Vaid N. Invisalign treatment with mandibular advancement: a retrospective cohort cephalometric appraisal. J Clin Imaging Sci. 2022;12:42.
2. Ravera S, Castroflorio T, Galati F, Cugliari G, Garino F, Deregibus A, et al. Short term dentoskeletal effects of mandibular advancement clear aligners in class II growing patients. A prospective controlled study according to STROBE guidelines. Eur J Paediatr Dent. 2021;22(2):119–24.
3. Rongo R, Dianiskova S, Spiezia A, Bucci R, Michelotti A, D'Anto V. Class II malocclusion in adult patients: what are the effects of the Intermaxillary elastics with clear aligners? A retrospective single center one-group longitudinal study. J Clin Med. 2022;11(24):7333.
4. Koukou M, Damanakis G, Tsolakis AI. Orthodontic management of skeletal class II malocclusion with the Invisalign mandibular advancement feature appliance: a case report and review of the literature. Case Rep Dent. 2022;2022:7095467.
5. Theroux KL. A new vacuum-formed phase I retainer. J Clin Orthod. 2003;37(7):384–7.

12.1 Introduction

Given the surge in uptake of orthodontic cases treated with aligners, it was only a matter of time before orthognathic cases were also treated using this technique. Historically, all stages of orthodontic treatment including the pre-surgical, the surgical and the post-surgical phases have been managed with fixed appliances. This three-stage approach requires at least 18 to 24 months with the first phase being the longest phase to obtain full decompensation of the dentition and allow for the surgical corrective movements. The surgical and the post-surgical orthodontic phases are usually much shorter duration with the latter's purpose being that of detailing refining the occlusion further.

The indication for resorting to orthognathic surgery to correct a malocclusion is when the scope of orthodontic treatment doesn't suffice to address the features of the presenting malocclusion. This is normally the case when the primary aetiological factor of the malocclusion is skeletal. Other indications include sleep apnoea, cleft lip and palate, hemifacial microsomia, syndromes affecting the facial structures and post-traumatic malocclusions [1].

The reasons for undertaking an orthognathic pathway is to improve the functional and extra- and intraoral aesthetic aspects of a malocclusion [2].

In the case of Invisalign® by Align Technology, Inc. (Santa Clara, CA, USA), a specific request for A-P changes using a surgical simulation can be chosen in the stage 5 of the prescription stage. The software allows the visualisation of the dental changes to improve the inter arch coordination, followed by a single-shift stage at the end of the 3D projection.

A different approach to the more classical three-stage approach mentioned above is the surgery-first approach. As the name of the technique implies, any orthodontic treatment is carried out following the surgical correction. In the case of aligner treatment using Invisalign® the ClinCheck® Pro 6 allows the flexibility of

S. Abela, *Aligner Systems in Invisible Orthodontics*,
https://doi.org/10.1007/978-3-031-49204-4_12

both approaches as the surgical movement can be placed at the start of the ClinCheck®, during treatment or towards the end. This allows the clinician the ability to plan the case based on the clinical presentation rather than being limited on a software application.

12.2   Efficacy of Aligners for Surgical Cases

Scientific evidence regarding the efficacy of aligners in treating surgical cases as opposed to using conventional appliances has now started to emerge and is available to the wider scientific community.

The efficiency of Invisalign® in managing surgical cases clinically has been reported numerous times. Case reports describing the processes involved in correcting malocclusions that require surgical correction are available including skeletal class III surgical cases [3, 4]. The efficiency of Invisalign® has also been described for most surgical interventions, including single jaw surgery and bimaxillary surgery [5, 6] and could be a very valid alternative to more traditional fixed appliances [7].

A comparison between fixed appliances and Invisalign® to manage surgical cases orthodontically is also available [8].

The true efficiency of tooth movement using clear aligners, specifically with Invisalign®, during the decompensation phase of the pre-surgical orthodontics has been measured at 63.4%. The lowest and highest average efficiency figures were 51.9% and 74.9%, respectively [9]. It was clear that certain mandibular tooth movements proved to be less efficient and this was valid for mesialisation in comparison to distalisation of molars, extrusion as opposed to intrusion and buccal torque as opposed to lingual torque.

12.3   Objectives of Aligners Pre-surgery

The objectives and aims of clear aligners, in line with other types of appliances including labial fixed appliances and lingual fixed appliances is to decompensate the dentition within the upper and lower arches. This equates to the complete reversal of any compensation that has occurred to camouflage the underlying skeletal base. In the upper arch, the upper incisors angulation to the maxillary base should be an average of 109° ± 6° whilst the lower incisors angulation to the mandibular base should be an average of 93° ± 6°.

The aims also include coordination of the arches to allow very good interdigitation between the maxillary and mandibular arches. This is obtained by eliminating any transverse discrepancies. The occlusal planes should also be levelled.

Once the above objectives are met, the clinicians should be able to obtain pre-surgical study models and replicate the post-surgery position of the two arches in occlusion. This certifies readiness to proceed with the planned jaw surgery.

12.4 Objectives of Aligners During Surgery or in the Immediate Postoperative Stage

This phase of treatment, without any doubt could present as the most difficult for the clinician. Traditionally, the patient proceeds to the jaw surgery procedure by having custom-made surgical splints produced. These can be easily secured to the fixed appliances during the surgical intervention. The role of surgical splints is well established in orthognathic surgery. They are key to providing very precise surgical jaw movements by relaying three main functions to the surgeon:

(a) They allow precise positioning of the maxilla and mandible relative to one another by adhering to the agreed planned position prior to the surgery.
(b) They prevent any unwanted sliding movements during intermaxillary fixation.
(c) They aid stabilisation of the new occlusion during intermaxillary fixation and post-surgery.

In case of aligners, this is not possible and other means of securing the surgical splints has to be sought. The options of securing the surgical splints also referred to as surgical wafers are as follows:

- Transitioning to labial or lingual fixed appliances just prior to and during the immediate post-surgery phase.
- Placement of arch bars to both arches.
- Placement of intermaxillary fixation (IMF) screws or orthodontic mini-implants (OMIs) also referred to as mini-screws.
- A combination of arch bars and mini-implants with the use of Stryker SMARTLock™ Hybrid MMF™.

12.5 Objectives of Aligners Post-surgery

The post-surgical phase could also pose a difficult phase to manage for the clinician. The difficulties arise mainly due to the inability to retake the dental impressions or digital scan for the post-surgical batch of aligners. Postoperatively the patient typically presents with very limited mouth opening and facial swelling with generalised tenderness of the oral structures.

The two possible ways of managing this stage is as follows:

(a) Taking the dental impressions or digital scan just prior to the surgery. This has the potential disadvantage of not being able to fully anticipate the precise position of the teeth or occlusion postoperatively.
(b) Taking dental impressions or digital scans postoperatively. This is usually not possible before 2 months postoperatively due to the reasons mentioned above with the added disadvantage that unwanted tooth movement might have occurred.

References

1. Larsen MK. Indications for orthognathic surgery—A review. Oral Health Dent Manag. 2017;2017:1–13.
2. Cremona M, Bister D, Sheriff M, Abela S. Quality-of-life improvement, psychosocial benefits, and patient satisfaction of patients undergoing orthognathic surgery: a summary of systematic reviews. Eur J Orthod. 2022;44(6):603–13.
3. Marcuzzi E, Galassini G, Procopio O, Castaldo A, Contardo L. Surgical-Invisalign treatment of a patient with class III malocclusion and multiple missing teeth. J Clin Orthod. 2010;44(6):377–84.
4. Pagani R, Signorino F, Poli PP, Manzini P, Panisi I. The use of Invisalign(R) system in the management of the orthodontic treatment before and after class III surgical approach. Case Rep Dent. 2016;2016:9231219.
5. Womack WR, Day RH. Surgical-orthodontic treatment using the Invisalign system. J Clin Orthod. 2008;42(4):237–45.
6. Zhang W, Yang H. Orthognathic surgery in Invisalign patients. J Craniofac Surg. 2022;33(2):e112–e3.
7. Miranda SL, Oliveira MR, Cheim Junior AP, Moreno R, Miranda MVF, Barbosa RLL. Clear aligners combined with orthognathic surgery: a case series. Gen Dent. 2023;71(1):66–70.
8. Kankam H, Madari S, Sawh-Martinez R, Bruckman KC, Steinbacher DM. Comparing outcomes in orthognathic surgery using clear aligners versus conventional fixed appliances. J Craniofac Surg. 2019;30(5):1488–91.
9. Cong A, Ruellas ACO, Tai SK, Loh CT, Barkley M, Yatabe M, et al. Presurgical orthodontic decompensation with clear aligners. Am J Orthod Dentofacial Orthop. 2022;162(4):538–53.

Clinical Management of Hybrid Approaches with Aligners and Fixed Appliances, Sectional Lingual Appliances and Mini-implants

13

13.1 Introduction

The progress and modernisation that clear aligners have bestowed to the profession in conjunction with CAD-CAM technology is undeniable. Presented initially as an alternative to removable appliances for extremely mild cases and best-suited for single tooth movements, nowadays clear aligners are advocated for the most complex of cases. It is also undeniable however, that predicting treatment outcomes can be difficult. Equally, obtaining specific tooth movements with ease decreases proportionately to the perceived difficulty of a case.

It has been widely approved that one way of overcoming limitations of aligners is to combine them with other appliances. This approach, referred to as hybrid approach, increases a clinician's scope of practice and provides the patient with better outcomes at the end of treatment.

Clear aligners offer less predictability with specific tooth movements. These include extrusive and intrusive movements, expansion of the buccal segments, derotations, traction of upper lateral incisors and root movements including translation and torque. Over prescribing is usually recommended for these tooth movements; however, the hybrid approach is aimed at addressing these limitations and rendering aligners as versatile as possible. This should subsequently decrease the reliance on multiple refinement stages.

13.2 Overcoming Transverse Expansion Limitations

In traditional fixed appliance therapy, one of the commonest modalities of correcting the transverse discrepancies is with the application of expansion devices. These include removable appliances with midline expansion screws, quad-helix appliances and rapid maxillary expansion (RME) devices. The clinician's preferred method is solely based on the individual's requirements and the amount of correction needed. The most commonly used parameter to measure the transverse

© The Author(s), under exclusive license to Springer Nature Switzerland AG 2024
S. Abela, *Aligner Systems in Invisible Orthodontics*,
https://doi.org/10.1007/978-3-031-49204-4_13

Table 13.1 Choice of expansion device based on the degree of transpalatal discrepancy between the maxillary and the mandibular arches

Transpalatal width deficiency between the maxillary and mandibular arches	Treatment modalities of choice
Less than 1.5 mm	No indication for expansion
Between 1.5 and 2 mm	Fixed Archwire Expansion
Between 2 and 4 mm	Option 1. Removable appliances with midline expansion screw Option 2. Activated transpalatal arch Option 3. Quad-Helix appliance
Between 4 and 12 mm	TBRME—Tooth-Borne Rapid Maxillary Expansion BBRME—Bone-Borne Rapid Maxillary Expansion
More than 12 mm	SARME—Surgically Assisted RME

deficiency between the maxillary and mandibular arches is by measuring the transpalatal widths of the two arches. The most common landmark used is the mesio-buccal cusp due to its ease of being measured clinically. The indications for the use of the different types of expansion devices based on previously published recommendations is tabulated in Table 13.1 below [1].

With previously claimed efficiencies for transverse correction between 72.8% and 87.7% for the maxillary and mandibular arches, respectively, mostly achieved by tipping mechanisms, the hybrid approach be a natural fit for the aligner technique [2]. Predictability figures based the type of tooth under consideration, the range varied between 74.8% for canines, 80.3% and 81% for first and second premolars, respectively, and 79.1% and 65.2% for first and second molars, respectively [3]. Such an approach would therefore enable clinicians to provide patients with a separate expansion stage prior to the definitive aligner stage. The correction of the transverse dimension would decrease the duration of aligner wear and significantly increase the predictability of the final outcome.

13.3   Overcoming Rotational Movement Limitations

One of the least predictable tooth movements remains de-rotational movements for all teeth and most especially canines and premolars. This is thought to be due to the anatomical morphology disallowing efficient transmission of forces to the crown. One study measured the overall efficiency rate at 59% with an overall mean efficiency for premolar de-rotation even lower at 40% [4].

The clinician's hybrid approach in cases presenting with canine and/or premolar rotations should thus consider a hybrid approach. A phase of fixed appliances or sectional fixed appliances specifically intended to correct the rotations would also improve final outcomes and decrease the reliance on multiple refinement stages.

13.4 Combining Aligners with Orthodontic Mini-implants

The use of orthodontic mini-implants (OMIs) have increased the scope of orthodontics significantly, and this is equally valid for treatments carried out with aligners. The main indications of combining OMIs with aligners are as follows:

- Mesialisation or distilisation of buccal segments
- Correction of maxillary transverse deficiency
- Camouflage of class II malocclusions
- Indirect anchorage reinforcement
- Intrusion of buccal segments for:

  (a) the correction of anterior open bites
  (b) pre-prosthetic replacement of missing teeth

- Overbite reduction
- Molar uprighting
- Alignment of impacted teeth

13.4.1 Mesialisation or Distilisation of Buccal Segments with Aligners Orthodontic Mini-implants

Orthodontic mini-implants (OMIs) can be used very effectively for mesialisation or distalisation of the buccal segments.

13.4.1.1 Buccal Segment Mesialisation

The two most common indications for this type of biomechanics are the following:

- Mesialisation of one or two molars following the previous loss of a molar due to the restorative failure
- Hypodontia cases affecting the labial segments

The first or second molars are commonly extracted due to the lack of feasibility of restoring them or following failure of restorative treatment. The resultant edentulous site can be restored with mesial movement of the more distally placed molar [5].

In case of hypodontia cases, the most common scenarios are a missing upper lateral incisor ipsilaterally or naturally occurring missing upper lateral incisors bilaterally. In these cases, the ideal treatment plan would involve approximating the upper canines towards the central incisors with projection of the premolars and molars mesially without altering the position nor loss of any torque of all the teeth in the labial segment. This can be done by placing an OMI distal to the upper canines used as upper lateral incisor substitutes and using the OMIs to offer traction to the buccal segments [6]. Alternatively, the OMIs can be attached to a mesial slider and the aligner phase of treatment provided concomitantly or subsequently [7].

13.4.1.2   Buccal Segment Distalisation

Effectively the opposite mechanics to the above is the distalisation of the buccal segments. The indications for these mechanics would include:

- Altering the canine relationship to a class I
- Altering the molar relationship to a class I
- Camouflaging a class II malocclusion
- Pre-prosthetic placement of an implant by obtaining the required amount of interdental spacing

Distalisation of buccal segments is not only limited to the upper arch. Mandibular molars can also be distalised using OMIs to relieve crowding [8].

13.4.2 Correction of Maxillary Transverse Deficiency with Aligners Orthodontic Mini-implants

The use of OMIs to obtain palatal expansion is a very well-known technique. Combining it with aligners could render the entire treatment very indiscreet. The first stage of the treatment as described in Sect. 15.2 below could be dedicated to the correction of the transverse deficiency followed by the provision of the definitive aligners. The OMI-based expansion devices, although very similar in design to conventional expansion appliances, are completely bone-borne. The placement of the OMIs is in the midline section of the palate posterior to the palatal rugae on either side of the mid-palatal suture. A vast amount of literature about this technique including case reports, clinical trials, and textbooks are available that describe the procedure in much more detail. The aligners would then be utilised as a second stage of treatment following the transverse correction which would not be the most efficient movement obtainable by the aligners.

13.4.3 Camouflaging Class II Malocclusions with Aligners and Orthodontic Mini-implants

Class II malocclusions often present with a more mesial projection of the maxillary arch in comparison with the mandibular arch. This is often the case with the canine and molar relationship.

Obtaining class I canines and molar relationship can be achieved with aligners by prescribing buccal segment distalisation, and this type of mechanics records the highest amount of efficiency. A predictable amount of molar distalisation with aligners would range between 2 and 3 mm [8, 9, 10]. In a very recent study, the accuracy of distilisation was proven to be higher for second maxillary molars at 75% in comparison to the maxillary first molars at 69% [11]. Other studies could quote greater efficacy rates for this type of movement with rates reaching 87% [12].

The advantages of using OMIs in conjunction to aligners would be twofold:

1. Increase the scope achieving greater amounts of distalisation.

   - For the maxillary arch: The OMI placement can be either in the maxillary tuberosity [13] or on either side of the mid-palatal suture and connected to a distalising device such as the Beneslider [14, 15].

2. Prevent anchorage loss by preventing proclination of upper incisors during the distalisation phase. With distalisation techniques the clinician can only expect a reactionary affect on the incisors which could only manifest with increased protrusion if anchorage is not controlled. One of the ways of controlling this is via the use of class II inter arch elastics or with the use of OMIs.

13.4.4 Provision of Indirect Anchorage with Aligners and Orthodontic Mini-implants

OMIs can be used in both the maxillary and mandibular arches to reinforce anchorage. This allows more difficult tooth movements to be achieved more successfully with or without the concomitant use of aligners. The indirect application of OMI aims to reduce the movement of any anchorage units used in biomechanics.
Examples of such use include the following placements:
In the maxillary arch:

- Mid-palatal suture placement with attachment to the palatal aspect of the upper incisors for mesial traction of canines and/or premolars.
- Buccal placement between the second premolar and the first molar with attachment to the archwire to allow traction to the labial segment for retraction.
- Posterior palatal placement for the traction of impacted canines.

   In the mandibular arch:

- Buccal placement between the lateral incisor and the canine or between the canine and the first premolar with attachment to the archwire.
- Buccal placement with ligation to one tooth to provide traction to an adjacent tooth for mesial or distal traction.

13.4.5 Intrusion of Buccal segments with Aligners and Orthodontic Mini-implants

Intrusion of buccal segments with OMIs is a very well-known technique. This procedure can be applied before the definitive aligner treatment or could be applied at the same time during the aligner process.
Intrusion can be achieved via elastomeric attachments or by being applied on the aligner.

13.4.6 Overbite Reduction with Aligners and Orthodontic Mini-implants

OMIs can be easily used ideally in tandem with the aligner treatment by placing them bilaterally in the sulcus region of the labial segment. This can be done either in the maxillary, mandibular arch or both. The main intention would be to obtain intrusion in the labial segment en masse rather than individual intrusion.

13.4.7 Molar Uprighting with Aligners and Orthodontic Mini-implants

Molar uprighting with OMIs is an additional benefit of incorporating them into the biomechanics. Aligners are not very effective at this type of movement due to the type of movement needed. This is equally valid whether attachments are utilised or not. Given that tipping is the main and most successful movement used by aligners, this mechanism would be very taxing on molars especially if a molar is not lone-standing but the more distal molars are present.

13.4.8 Alignment of Impacted Teeth with Aligners and Orthodontic Mini-implants

Aligner treatment is also much more complex and more demanding on the clinician when a case presents with impacted teeth. In such cases, applying OMIs could be extremely advantageous as they can be used to apply traction to the impacted tooth without involving any of the other teeth in the arch.

A typical example is with maxillary impacted canines where OMIs can be placed in the molar region and elastomeric attachments can be placed directly between the OMI and the impacted canines. The aligners in this case can be aimed at providing different biomechanics altogether decreasing the treatment duration for the benefit of the patient undergoing treatment.

13.5 Combining Aligners with Lingual Fixed Orthodontic Appliances

An excellent description in the form of a case report of how these two appliances, lingual fixed appliances and aligners has been given in the literature by Lombardo et al. 2020 [16]. The description of the ideal use of lingual fixed appliances in tandem with aligners was to improve the deficiency in certain tooth movements. In this specific case report, the utilisation of the lingual appliances has been used for the alignment of a buccally displaced canine in the upper arch and to de-rotate a premolar in the lower arch. This hybrid approach has been described by the author as a means of decreasing treatment time with an added advantage of the aligner covering the lingual attachments and adding additional comfort to the patient without resorting to comfort wax.

References

1. Bishara SE. Textbook of orthodontics. Elsevier (A Division of Reed Elsevier India Pvt. Limited); 2001.
2. Houle JP, Piedade L, Todescan R Jr, Pinheiro FH. The predictability of transverse changes with Invisalign. Angle Orthod. 2017;87(1):19–24.
3. Morales-Burruezo I, Gandia-Franco JL, Cobo J, Vela-Hernandez A, Bellot-Arcis C. Arch expansion with the Invisalign system: efficacy and predictability. PLoS One. 2020;15(12):e0242979.
4. Simon M, Keilig L, Schwarze J, Jung BA, Bourauel C. Treatment outcome and efficacy of an aligner technique—regarding incisor torque, premolar derotation and molar distalization. BMC Oral Health. 2014;14:68.
5. Palone M, Casella S, De Sbrocchi A, Siciliani G, Lombardo L. Space closure by miniscrew-assisted mesialization of an upper third molar and partial vestibular fixed appliance: a case report. Int Orthod. 2022;20(1):100602.
6. Wilmes B, Schwarze J, Vasudavan S, Drescher D. Maxillary space closure using aligners and palatal mini-implants in patients with congenitally missing lateral incisors. J Clin Orthod. 2021;55(1):20–33.
7. Wilmes B, Nienkemper M, Nanda R, Lubberink G, Drescher D. Palatally anchored maxillary molar mesialization using the mesialslider. J Clin Orthod. 2013;47(3):172–9.
8. Auladell A, De La Iglesia F, Quevedo O, Walter A, Puigdollers A. The efficiency of molar distalization using clear aligners and mini-implants: two clinical cases. Int Orthod. 2022;20(1):100604.
9. Ravera S, Castroflorio T, Garino F, Daher S, Cugliari G, Deregibus A. Maxillary molar distalization with aligners in adult patients: a multicenter retrospective study. Prog Orthod. 2016;17:12.
10. Saif BS, Pan F, Mou Q, Han M, Bu W, Zhao J, et al. Efficiency evaluation of maxillary molar distalization using Invisalign based on palatal rugae registration. Am J Orthod Dentofacial Orthop. 2022;161(4):e372–e9.
11. D'Anto V, Valletta R, Ferretti R, Bucci R, Kirlis R, Rongo R. Predictability of maxillary molar distalization and derotation with clear aligners: a prospective study. Int J Environ Res Public Health. 2023;20(4):2941.
12. Verma P, George AM. Efficacy of clear aligners in producing molar distalization: systematic review. APOS Trends Orthod. 2022;11:317–24.
13. Sada Garralda VJ. Simultaneous intrusion and distalization using miniscrews in the maxillary tuberosity. J Clin Orthod. 2016;50(10):605–12.
14. Wilmes B, Nienkemper M, Ludwig B, Kau CH, Pauls A, Drescher D. Esthetic class II treatment with the Beneslider and aligners. J Clin Orthod. 2012;46(7):390–8; quiz 437.
15. Wilmes B, Nanda R, Nienkemper M, Ludwig B, Drescher D. Correction of upper-arch asymmetries using the Mesial-Distalslider. J Clin Orthod. 2013;47(11):648–55.
16. Lombardo L, Palone M, Carlucci A, Siciliani G. Clear aligner hybrid approach: a case report. J World Fed Orthod. 2020;9(1):32–43.

Part III

Clinical Tips and Techniques to Aligner Therapy

Limitations of Aligner Applications

14.1 Introduction

Invisalign®, launched in 1998, has captured the attention of a wide range of clinicians including both specialist and non-specialist dental professionals. With its roots tracing back to Kesling's original positioner, followed by Ponitz's and Sheridan's introduction of the IPR technique, aligners have improved in their delivery and outcomes. Since their introduction various add-ons, also known as auxiliaries, have rendered the appliances more efficient. The ultimate aim for both the manufacturers and the clinicians is to continuously improve the efficacy of the appliances however persistent reported deficiencies include the following:

- Decreased efficiency in comparison to fixed appliances
- Decreased stability postoperatively
- The need to undertake multiple refinement stages
- The need to have a separate course of fixed appliance treatment to improve outcomes
- Decreased satisfactory occlusal outcomes
- Decreased control of crown-root movement
- Inaccuracies between predicted and achieved clinical outcomes

This chapter will also aim at expanding and giving further insights into these claimed deficiencies.

14.2 Decreased Efficiency in Comparison to Fixed Appliances

The perceived inferiority in delivering clinical efficiency in comparison to fixed appliances include the following:

© The Author(s), under exclusive license to Springer Nature Switzerland AG 2024
S. Abela, *Aligner Systems in Invisible Orthodontics*,
https://doi.org/10.1007/978-3-031-49204-4_14

- A lower average predictable outcome of 40% [1]
- A sub-optimal force delivery
- Decreased flexibility of the appliance
- Degradation of material over time
- A poor stress relaxation with a decay in force delivery most steep with 90% of force lost over the first 2 h
- Lack of appliance activation possibilities
- An associated and reliant AI that does not predict biological variables very accurately
- Degradation of material with exposure to the oral environment
- High deformation
- Low resilience
- High purchase point

14.3 Decreased Stability Postoperatively

An aspect of clear aligner treatment which is thought to be inferior to conventional fixed appliances is postoperative stability once treatment has been completed. This is a very important aspect if suspicions are raised that an appliance system is not able to maintain the desired tooth position postoperatively.

A study involving a systematic review analysing the available data suggests that stability is lower in patients that were treated with clear aligners [2].

One study utilising the ABO grading tool, with two main limitations in the study being segment of teeth analysed limited to upper labial segment and using removable retainers only, the group with CA experienced more relapse [3].

In cases requiring surgery, postoperative stability for patients that had undergone orthognathic surgery no differences could be noticed between the two types of systems. Moon et al. used both 2D and 3D radiographs to assess postoperative stability and two cohorts receiving fixed appliances and clear aligners were directly compared. No significant differences were found between the two groups in terms of postoperative stability.

The cohort receiving FA treatment had shorter pre-surgical phases of treatment; however, overall there were no differences between the two modalities [4].

14.4 The Need to Undertake Multiple Refinement Stages

The need of multiple refinement stages is taken as part and parcel of aligner treatment. Discrepancies between the digitised and the actual outcomes will lead to failure of trays to fit well over the whole course of treatment. An additional unfavourable outcome includes the successful attainment of the final tray with good fitting; however, the position of the teeth is less satisfactory.

This aspect of treatment can be considered as less efficacious than fixed appliance therapy as once they are fitted, aside from the occasional bracket breakage that the patient and the clinician experience there wouldn't be the need to add further appliances at the end of treatment. This could also be the reason why multiple authors of previous publications recommend aligners for mild to moderate cases but need to be avoided for more complex cases. For most clear aligner treatments, one set of aligners is thus the exception and not the norm [5].

14.5 The Need to Have a Separate Course of Fixed Appliance Treatment to Improve Outcomes

It is commonplace amongst users of clear aligners to use fixed appliances as an adjunct to improve the clinical outcomes. This decision is based on the presenting malocclusion and the clinician aware of the shortcomings of aligner treatment attempts at overcoming these with the introduction of fixed appliances.

14.6 Decreased Satisfactory Occlusal Outcomes

Fixed appliances are superior to clear aligners at postoperative occlusal outcomes. A study analysing this specifically used the Peer Assessment Rating (PAR) index, a quantitative measure to assess postoperative orthodontic outcome. The authors found that in general, pretreatment PAR score of fixed appliances is higher than that of clear aligners representing management of malocclusions with higher complexities are treated with fixed appliances. The post-treatment score is also lower in the aligner group representing a poorer clinical outcome when compared to the fixed appliances group [6].

14.7 Decreased Control of Crown-Root Movement

It could be considered a difficult movement in orthodontics in general, however accomplishing this type of movement with clear aligners could even be more difficult than with fixed appliances.

The clinician should be aware that this movement is possible with aligners albeit with much less efficacy than the software might suggest and with the use of the correct type of attachments [7].

14.8 Inaccuracies Between Predicted and Achieved Clinical Outcomes

As evidenced in previous chapters and paragraphs, aligners undoubtedly provided a change in the provision of orthodontics. One aspect that remains unclear and difficult to quantify is the precision between the predicted result simulated on the ClinCheck Pro® software and the real-life outcomes. The precise validity of the software and its correlation with live movements remains to be defined accurately. A study aiming at quantifying this found that the software is inaccurate at representing the actual movements that took place during the treatment phase. The authors also found exaggerations in the predicted movements [8]. The findings of another study were in agreement with regard to the imprecision at overbite management but Invisalign® was accurate at predicting the other type of tooth movements [9].

Additional and more contemporary studies specifically looking at the accuracy with expansion movements in both the maxilla and mandible were found to be 72.8% and 87.7% accurate [10]. The authors recommended the need to prescribe overexpansion movements to accomplish the desired outcomes and counteract the inaccuracies posed by the software prediction.

The efficiency in very recent studies suggest much lower precision and efficiency rates of 45% for both maxillary contraction and expansion [11]. This would be very much in line with a previously referenced study quoting 41% [1].

References

1. Kravitz ND, Kusnoto B, BeGole E, Obrez A, Agran B. How well does Invisalign work? A prospective clinical study evaluating the efficacy of tooth movement with Invisalign. Am J Orthod Dentofacial Orthop. 2009;135(1):27–35.
2. Kassam SK, Stoops FR. Are clear aligners as effective as conventional fixed appliances? Evid Based Dent. 2020;21(1):30–1.
3. Tamer I, Oztas E, Marsan G. Orthodontic treatment with clear aligners and the scientific reality behind their marketing: a literature review. Turk J Orthod. 2019;32(4):241–6.
4. Moon C, Sándor GK, Ko EC, Kim Y-D. Postoperative stability of patients undergoing orthognathic surgery with orthodontic treatment using clear aligners: a preliminary study. Appl Sci. 2021;11(23):11216.
5. Robertson L, Kaur H, Fagundes NCF, Romanyk D, Major P, Flores MC. Effectiveness of clear aligner therapy for orthodontic treatment: a systematic review. Orthod Craniofac Res. 2020;23(2):133–42.
6. Gu J, Tang JS, Skulski B, Fields HW Jr, Beck FM, Firestone AR, et al. Evaluation of Invisalign treatment effectiveness and efficiency compared with conventional fixed appliances using the peer assessment rating index. Am J Orthod Dentofacial Orthop. 2017;151(2):259–66.
7. Smith JM, Weir T, Kaang A, Farella M. Predictability of lower incisor tip using clear aligner therapy. Prog Orthod. 2022;23(1):37.
8. Buschang PH, Ross M, Shaw SG, Crosby D, Campbell PM. Predicted and actual end-of-treatment occlusion produced with aligner therapy. Angle Orthod. 2015;85(5):723–7.
9. Krieger E, Seiferth J, Marinello I, Jung BA, Wriedt S, Jacobs C, et al. Invisalign(R) treatment in the anterior region: were the predicted tooth movements achieved? J Orofac Orthop. 2012;73(5):365–76.
10. Houle JP, Piedade L, Todescan R Jr, Pinheiro FH. The predictability of transverse changes with Invisalign. Angle Orthod. 2017;87(1):19–24.
11. Riede U, Wai S, Neururer S, Reistenhofer B, Riede G, Besser K, et al. Maxillary expansion or contraction and occlusal contact adjustment: effectiveness of current aligner treatment. Clin Oral Investig. 2021;25(7):4671–9.

Overcoming Aligners' Limitations   15

15.1   Introduction

Upon consideration of the above-mentioned inherent aligner material deficiencies, the user could vary their biomechanics to accommodate these same deficiencies.

Once aligner treatment is under consideration, six biomechanical and treatment strategies can be applied to improve the outcomes of treatment. These are mentioned and described below.

15.2   Case Selection

It has been reported in the literature that aligners are much more efficient at treating more straightforward cases of malocclusion involving mild to moderate degrees of crowding [1]. Case selection remains a priority when considering clear aligners.

15.3   Predominant Tipping Movements

Tooth tipping is a much more readily accomplished type of tooth movement in comparison to more complex movement such as translation or root movement. Careful consideration should be given on the type of tooth movements required to obtain the intended outcomes to a case and ensure that the outcomes can be achieved predominantly with tipping movements. The aligner material properties allow shape-moulding and provide compressive forces over the entire tooth surface area resulting in predominantly tipping movement.

© The Author(s), under exclusive license to Springer Nature Switzerland AG 2024   129
S. Abela, *Aligner Systems in Invisible Orthodontics*,
https://doi.org/10.1007/978-3-031-49204-4_15

15.4   Programming Less Movement

With high deformation rates and poor stress-strain properties, programming less tooth movement in each aligner will expose these deficiencies less.

15.5   Extend Treatment Time

Although the patients' requests would always lean on making the treatment as short as possible, in the case of aligner treatment, spreading the tooth movement over a larger number of trays will reduce tracking errors and the need to have multiple refinement stages. This is obtained by increasing the precision between the intended and actual tooth movement for each aligner.

15.6   Increase the Rate of Tray Change

By changing the trays more frequently the user will be making allowance for the force degradation that is very steep in the first 2 h. Rapid changing of trays will maintain consistency and precision with less chances of tracking issues propagating throughout the treatment duration.

15.7   Choice of Aligner System

The users' choice on the type of aligner system can be based on the material thickness provided by the manufacturer. The thicker the tray which can vary between 0.5 and 1.5 mm will provide varying degrees of forces with thinner trays providing lighter forces ideally for tipping movements whilst thicker trays will provide higher forces more suitable for translation or root movements.

Reference

1. Tamer I, Oztas E, Marsan G. Orthodontic treatment with clear aligners and the scientific reality behind their marketing: a literature review. Turk J Orthod. 2019;32(4):241–6.

Patient Motivation for Long-Term Compliance for Complex Treatments

16

16.1 Introduction

Analysis of the variation in compliance between genders during fixed appliance treatment has been well reported in the literature, with females being better than males at adhering to the instructions given. Other factors directly associated with increased compliance included the household socioeconomic status and parents' level of education attained at the time of treatment [1]. With the technological advancements at hand, compliance adherence can be monitored more closely however given the extreme range of ages that clear aligners (CA) might be catering for, the treating clinician should also expect a variation in compliance based on age differences. In case of fixed appliance therapy greater compliance and adherence with postoperative instructions has been observed, and this could be extrapolated to CA therapy [2].

In a specific study analysing factors that could affect compliance with CA therapy, the authors found that males were more likely to comply with the treatment however age and preconception of the patients' smiles played no part in affecting compliance. Patients that had previous orthodontic treatment were less likely to be compliant and vice versa [3].

16.2 Poor Compliance Indicators

Compliance as mentioned above is key to a treatment's success. Poor compliance can be directly associated with certain features, characteristics and previous patient experiences; however, the treating clinician should always remain vigilant against such a possibility.

Below are ten signs that could be a telltale sign of poor compliance:

1. Multiple missed appointments
2. Multiple lost aligners

© The Author(s), under exclusive license to Springer Nature Switzerland AG 2024
S. Abela, *Aligner Systems in Invisible Orthodontics*,
https://doi.org/10.1007/978-3-031-49204-4_16

3. Non-coordinated tray numbers between the upper and lower arches
4. Poorly fitting trays
5. Discrepancy between claimed hours of wear between patient and accompanying parents or partner
6. No discolouration of compliance indicator
7. Extremely clean aligners
8. Sealed packets with unworn aligners
9. Third parties booking future follow-up appointments
10. Cancelled appointments with no or very brief notice

16.3 Overcoming Poor Compliance

The following technologies and adjuncts aim at improving wear compliance and can be used individually or as a combination especially if compliance is anticipated.

16.3.1 Log Book

The concept of introducing a log book to log the number of hours of daily wear had been originally introduced for headgear devices. This technique was later adapted for functional appliances and later also applied for clear aligners.

The efficacy of recording the daily hours of headgear used increased the compliance and improved clinical outcomes.

16.3.2 Timers

Timers have in the past also been originally aimed at improving headgear compliance. Use of Compliance Science System (CSS) via the placement of an electric module in the headstrip have been shown to improve headgear wear by 4½–6 h per day [4]. Simpler timers used by Cureton et al. also showed improved compliance with headgear use [5]. In today's modern times, these timers have been replaced with apps that act as reminders however they can also be found with timer feature built-in.

16.3.3 Other Types of Technology

Other forms of technological aids that can improve compliance include the following:

1. Short Message Service (SMS)—The clinician can activate an automatic SMS service that reminds the patient to keep wearing the aligner for the amount of time provided in the postoperative instructions.

2. Emails—Emails can also be used as a form of reminder similarly to SMS, and emails can also have audiovisual aids to further strengthen the importance of wearing the aligners as recommended.
3. Remote monitoring Apps—Given the daily use of cellular devices computer and mobile apps form a very contemporary way of serving as a reminder and/or timer. Further details about technological apps can be found in Chap. 19 below.

16.3.4 Compliance Indicator

Based on historic findings with previous types of orthodontic appliances, Align Technology, Inc., also attempted at decreasing lack of compliance with its aligners. First introduced in Invisalign Teen® the compliance indicator was a blue circular spot embedded in the aligner to improve wear compliance in this age group. This indicator was also used for adult aligners.

Consisting of a dye, the aim of its placement is to demonstrate a good wear regimen over a 2-week period with a consistent level of fading between trays. The fading process commences with the first contact between the patient's saliva and the tray. Generally, the blue indicators are placed in the first molar region, and the fading gradually changes the dark blue dot into a clear one if the patient adhered to the recommended amount of wear.

Compliance indicators and their effectiveness were investigated in the past showing clinical effectiveness and a positive effect when used [6]. The clinician nevertheless has to remain vigilant on misuse of the compliance indicators mimicking the intraoral use as instructed by the clinician [7].

References

1. Al-Abdallah M, Hamdan M, Dar-Odeh N. Traditional vs digital communication channels for improving compliance with fixed orthodontic treatment. Angle Orthod. 2021;91(2):227–35.
2. Barbosa IV, Ladewig VM, Almeida-Pedrin RR, Cardoso MA, Santiago Junior JF, Conti A. The association between patient's compliance and age with the bonding failure of orthodontic brackets: a cross-sectional study. Prog Orthod. 2018;19(1):11.
3. Timm LH, Farrag G, Baxmann M, Schwendicke F. Factors influencing patient compliance during clear aligner therapy: a retrospective cohort study. J Clin Med. 2021;10(14):3103.
4. Doruk C, Agar U, Babacan H. The role of the headgear timer in extraoral co-operation. Eur J Orthod. 2004;26(3):289–91.
5. Cureton SL, Regennitter F, Orbell MG. An accurate, inexpensive headgear timer. J Clin Orthod. 1991;25(12):749–54.
6. Tuncay OC, Bowman SJ, Nicozisis JL, Amy BD. Effectiveness of a compliance indicator for clear aligners. J Clin Orthod. 2009;43(4):263–8; quiz 73–4
7. Schott TC, Goz G. Color fading of the blue compliance indicator encapsulated in removable clear Invisalign Teen(R) aligners. Angle Orthod. 2011;81(2):185–91.

3D Software Planning Considerations for Crown-Root Movements

17

17.1 Introduction

Align Technology, Inc., San Jose, California, USA claim that major tooth movements such as over 50° of de-rotation and incisor torque expression are realistic expectations from their aligners. These types of movements are difficult to accomplish and to date fixed appliances remain the gold standard at achieving them; however, advances have rendered such movements possible.

Invisalign® has been found in the past to be less than ideal at expressing the prescribed torque [1] and hence the reason for lingering doubt about the acclaimed possibilities suggested by the manufacturers [2]. The clinician's responsibility is to understand how best to achieve these movements and the most accurate way of achieving this.

The possibility of achieving the above-named movements with aligners was suggested in a study proving that body bodily movements and torque expression is possible [3]. The delivery of necessary forces and moments were successfully shown rendering the literature claims for obtaining these difficult movements accountable.

There are three main ways of obtaining torque during the prescription stage:

1. Power ridges
2. Attachments
3. Divots

The sections below provide further detail into these techniques separately.

© The Author(s), under exclusive license to Springer Nature Switzerland AG 2024

S. Abela, *Aligner Systems in Invisible Orthodontics*,

https://doi.org/10.1007/978-3-031-49204-4_17

17.2 Power Ridges

Power ridges (PRs) are a SmartForce® feature found on the gingival third of the buccal aspect of the Invisalign® aligners. Their inclusion in the prescription is solely for the delivery of torque expression most commonly lingual root torque to the upper or lower incisors. It is a default inclusion by the software if three or more degrees (3°) of incisor torque expression is needed.

PRs can be coupled with additional ridges on the lingual aspect of the Invisalign® aligners for additional efficacy. This feature usually added to complement the buccal power ridge is available on upper incisors. The main indication for prescribing buccal PR in contrast to buccal and lingual PRs is when torque to the incisors is needed only. If torque and retraction form part of the movements in the clinician's treatment plan, both types of PRs will be needed. As mentioned before, the threshold for inclusion within the prescription is 3° of torque with 1° of change per tray.

In study carried out specifically designed to look at the efficacy of power ridges (PRs) in producing torque of more than 10° in the upper labial segment, no difference in torque expression was produced by the PRs when compared to the recommended ellipsoid attachment [4]. In the same study, the recommended horizontal ellipsoid attachments were also analysed for efficiency. The overall efficacy of tooth movement in the study was recorded at 59.3%, and it also included observations on premolar de-rotations and molar distalisation and not on the overall efficacy of orthodontic tooth movement. In the case of the latter, this type of movement proved to be the most difficult tooth movement to accomplish, and hence the association of this movement with the lowest efficacy measured at 23.6%. No difference was found with and without the use of an attachment.

Direct comparison of PRs to horizontal ellipsoid attachments showed no significant differences. Mean accuracies for the former compared to the latter were 51.5% and 49.1%. The highest and lowest accuracies recorded were 75.1% and 27.4% for the PR group and 71.6% and 29.9% for the attachment group showing very similar extremes of accuracies at both extremes.

The outcomes achieved by horizontal ellipsoid attachments were very different in a separate study using finite element analysis finding them superior than PRs and to not having any auxiliaries [5].

Positive outcomes were also observed by another group of authors demonstrating good outcomes when torque of less than 10° was needed [6].

17.3 Attachments

Attachments as recommended by the manufacturer to actuate torque have to be horizontal ellipsoid with a bevel on the gingival aspect of the attachment. Additional details about the variations in shape of attachments can be found in Chap. 3.

17.4 Divots

Divots are clinically placed pressure points applied by the clinician with the use of aligner pliers. These pressure points are aimed at creating a force couple resulting in torque with root movement in the desired direction. The divots are placed strategically depending on the type of movement required.

For lingual root torque, two divots are placed: one on the gingival third of the buccal aspect of the aligner and a synergistic divot on the incisal third of the aligner on the lingual aspect.

For buccal root torque, two divots are placed in an opposite manner: one divot is placed on the gingival third of the lingual surface of the aligner and the second divot is placed on the buccal aspect of the incisor one-third of the aligner. Figure 17.1 below illustrates the divot placement principle, whilst Fig. 17.2 illustrates the clinical application. The straight arrows in the illustration depict the forces created whilst the curvaceous arrows depict the resultant torque expression.

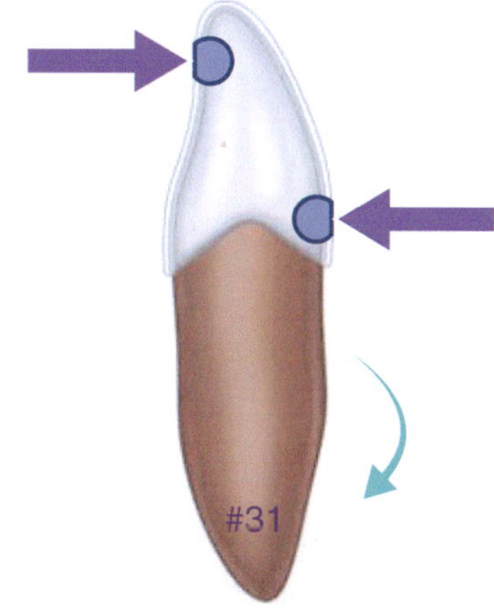

Fig. 17.1 Two synergistic divots placed for lingual root torque. This image has been reproduced from JCO 2020

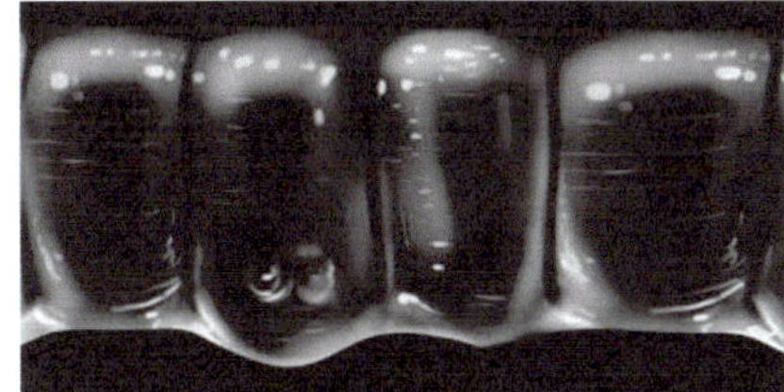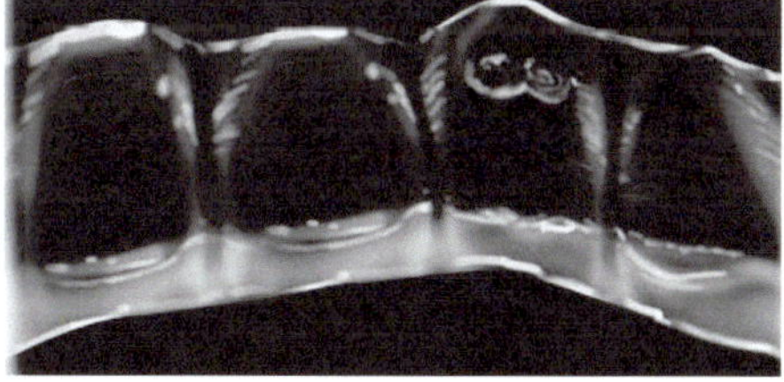

Fig. 17.2 Clinical divot placement on an aligner for lingual root torque of lower left central incisor. This image has been reproduced from JCO 2020

References

1. Gu J, Tang JS, Skulski B, Fields HW Jr, Beck FM, Firestone AR, et al. Evaluation of Invisalign treatment effectiveness and efficiency compared with conventional fixed appliances using the peer assessment rating index. Am J Orthod Dentofacial Orthop. 2017;151(2):259–66.
2. Brezniak N. The clear plastic appliance: a biomechanical point of view. Angle Orthod. 2008;78(2):381–2.
3. Simon M, Keilig L, Schwarze J, Jung BA, Bourauel C. Forces and moments generated by removable thermoplastic aligners: incisor torque, premolar derotation, and molar distalization. Am J Orthod Dentofacial Orthop. 2014;145(6):728–36.
4. Simon M, Keilig L, Schwarze J, Jung BA, Bourauel C. Treatment outcome and efficacy of an aligner technique—regarding incisor torque, premolar derotation and molar distalization. BMC Oral Health. 2014;14:68.
5. Sandhya V, Arun A, Reddy VP, Mahendra S, Chandrashekar B, Aravind. Biomechanical effects of Torquing on upper central incisor with thermoplastic aligner: a comparative three-dimensional finite element study with and without Auxillaries. J Indian Orthod Soc. 2022;56(1):49–56.
6. Castroflorio T, Garino F, Lazzaro A, Debernardi C. Upper-incisor root control with Invisalign appliances. J Clin Orthod. 2013;47(6):346–51; quiz 87

Clinical Tips for Treatment and Finishing

18

18.1 Introduction

Intraoral features that can be considered challenging to a clinician could invariably cause inconsistent finishing results and outcomes. These include, tooth rotations, tooth-size discrepancies, anterior and/or posterior crossbites, tooth inclination and torque expression.

IPR can also be considered challenging especially with regards to timing of this technique for the individual patient that is under treatment.

The sub-sections below provide a description of the frequently applicable tips and techniques that can be easily adopted when using clear aligners.

18.2 Clinical Tip for Correction of Molar Rotations

The first molars' rotational tendency has been in the past, measured to be present in the majority of the cases; 83% in all malocclusions and with an even greater majority in Class II division 1 malocclusions, 95% [1].

Rotated teeth occupy more space within an arch and consequentially aligning them will result in space gain [2]. This is usually 1 mm per molar and thus the space gain is 2 mm per arch. De-rotation of molars is also directly associated with distal movement and thus alteration of the molar relationship. This is equivalent to approximately 10° of molar de-rotation [3]. This characteristic molar eruptive pathway being with a more mesial positioning is correlated and could be exacerbated due to the following anatomical and occlusal traits:

- The rhomboidal anatomical crown of a first permanent molar [4]
- The availability of the leeway space resulting from the dimensional reduction between primary second molars and second premolars [5]
- Rotation around the larger but single palatal root [6]

© The Author(s), under exclusive license to Springer Nature Switzerland AG 2024
S. Abela, *Aligner Systems in Invisible Orthodontics*,
https://doi.org/10.1007/978-3-031-49204-4_18

- Early loss of second primary molars due to the decay [6]
- Jaw-tooth size discrepancies especially marked in class II malocclusions [1]

In fixed appliance therapy, this could be addressed with an active transpalatal arch and similarly in clear aligner technique the prescription can include de-rotation of the molars. The space gained with this movement can be used to:

1. Maintain the space gained for additional alignment within the arch [7].
2. Correct the buccal segment relationship [8].
3. Facilitate additional buccal segment distalisation due to gain in arch perimeter [8].
4. Improve the interdigitation between the upper and lower arches [9].

18.3   Attachment Tips for Correction of Molar Rotations

Additional clinical tips that can be considered include the type of attachment placed on molars.

In cases where attachment on molars is considered for retention purposes only, ellipsoid attachments would be the attachment type of choice.

In cases where molar de-rotation is being planned with extrusive or intrusive movements, optimised multi-planar attachments will be the attachment type of choice.

In cases where transverse expansion is indicated in the upper molar area, horizontal attachments should be selected. The horizontal attachments will allow expansion without a loss of the buccolingual inclination and prevention of palatal cusps causing interocclusal interferences. The horizontal attachments can be bevelled gingival for added extrusive movements and bevelled occlusal if intrusive movement is needed simultaneously.

If distalisation movement of the molars is also needed, the attachment can be bevelled on the side where the molars need to be distalised to.

Attachments in the ClinCheck Pro® 6 can be added by dragging the attachment from the tool bar menu and dropping it on the selected tooth surface. The position, angulation and shape of the attachment can be altered digitally with the cursor. Refer to Fig. 18.1 to visualise the inclusion of a digital attachment. A blue circular arrow allows the user to change the angulation, the green arrow varies the prominence of the attachment whilst the red arrow modifies the bevel. Refer to Fig. 18.2a–c to visualise these modifications below.

The size of the attachment can also be varied by right clicking the mouse pad cursor and options of 1 mm incremental increases can be selected ranging from 3 to 5 mm or removing the attachment altogether. Figure 18.3 below shows the possibility of altering the attachment dimensions.

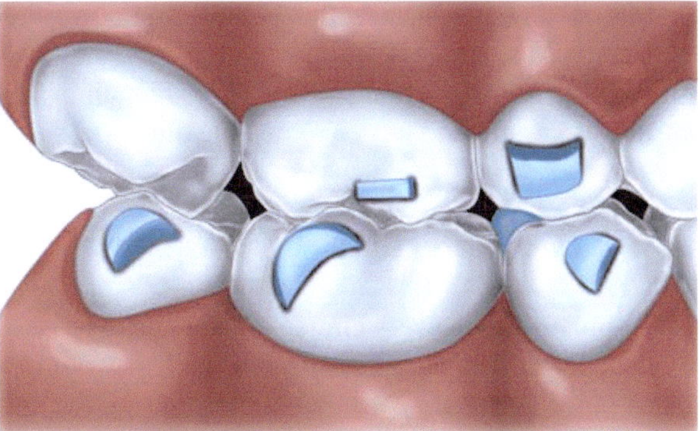

Fig. 18.1 Visual representation of an attachment inclusion digitally on an upper right first molar. The attachment being transitionally added appears in a different red hue to the other established attachments. The colour will be homogenous once the attachment position is finalised

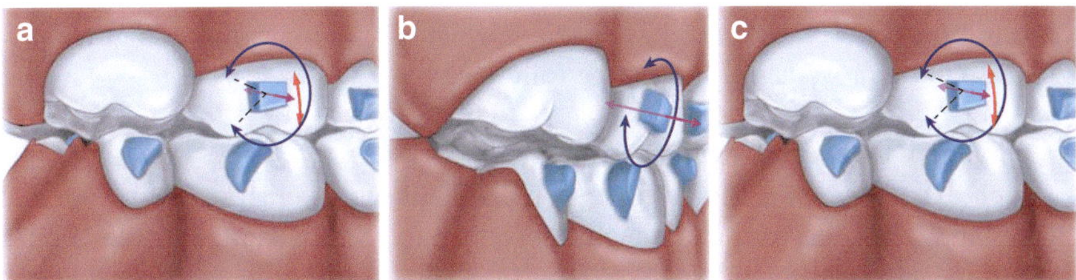

Fig. 18.2 (**a**), (**b**) and (**c**) allow visualisation of the blue, green and red arrows during inclusion a new attachment on the upper right first molar

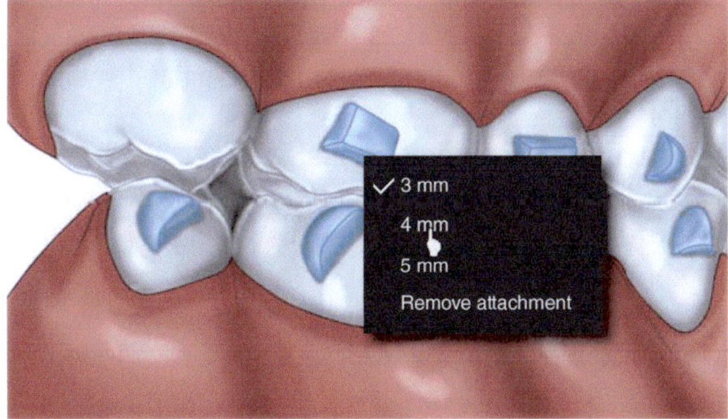

Fig. 18.3 Digital manipulation of an upper molar attachment size

18.4   Sequence of Tooth Movements for Maximal A-P Buccal Segment Correction

In order to obtain the best sagittal correction of the buccal segments, sequential molar distalisation technique should be applied to the stages following completion of upper molar de-rotation. Once all the de-rotation movements have been accomplished with the accompanying molar relationship changes, the user can analyse the need for further distalisation for full molar correction to class I.

Buccal segment distalisation is not only a very reliable tooth movement with aligners with a predictability as high as 88% but also very achievable with distal movements of up to 2 mm [10, 11, 12]. Maintaining these range of movements will ensure successful and more predictable outcomes.

18.5   Overcorrections

The ultimate aim of every clinician would be to reduce the need or resort to the least amount of refinement stages as possible. This would render the patients' experience much more satisfactory without compromising the planned outcome.

The above-mentioned ideal outcomes might necessitate the submission of prescriptions including overcorrections for some tooth movements. This is especially valid for tooth movements that have been associated with low efficacy figures.

These tooth movements include the following:

- **Maxillary transverse expansion**:
  Arch expansion is not fully expressed clinically with scientific estimations of 79.1% [13]. Other estimates include slightly reduced accuracy rate at 72.1% [14]. In addition, the constrictive effects of intermaxillary elastics on the arch won't be predicted successfully with the software's AI.
- **De-rotational movements**:
  The efficacy of aligners to accomplish de-rotatory movements has been repeatedly measured as low with previously conducted studies estimating the efficacy to be 40% [11]. This is also applicable for cases that present with bilaterally winged central incisors with mesio-palatal rotations affecting both central incisors [15].
- **Extrusive tooth movements**:
  Accuracy measurements for incisors extrusion was estimated at 56% whilst extrusion for mandibular molars was lower at 37% [16]. These figures would be considered low.
- **Intrusive tooth movements**:
  Incisor intrusion was estimated to be 33% and 51% for incisors and molars, respectively [16].
- **Incisor root torque:**
  The upper incisor torque has been estimated to occur in less than half of the prescribed amount, 42% [11]. Invisalign® has been proven to be more effective at expressing torque in the lower incisors in a lingual direction [17]. It is advisable that monitoring of incisor root torque is carried out though the duration of treatment especially for extraction cases involving premolars. Prescription of power ridges and additional root torque should be taken into consideration.
- **Deep bite management:**
  Overbite reduction was estimated to be, similarly to the movements mentioned above, low with regard to efficacy. Previous estimates have measured the rate to be 39.2% [18].

The amounts of efficacy quoted above will help the clinician to estimate the amount of overcorrection needed. Taking maxillary transverse expansion as an example, the user would need to estimate that approximately three quarters of the prescribed movement will be expressed. If the total need for expansion amounts to 6 mm, the clinician should expect a real-life space gain of 4.5 mm and an overcorrection of 1.5–2 mm is advisable to decrease the burden of numerous refinement stages.

18.6 Identification of Tooth-Size Discrepancies

It is always advisable to localise the tooth-size discrepancy at the planning phase of treatment.

This is firstly done by:

1. Identifying the arch—If the discrepancy is found in the maxilla, it is referred to as maxillary excess whereas if it is found in the mandible, this is referred to mandibular excess.
2. Identifying the tooth/teeth discrepancy—Identifying larger or smaller crowns in mesio-distal widths will also guide the clinician to the amount and site of IPR needed.

The best method to identify tooth-size discrepancies is by utilising the Bolton's discrepancy formula. For further details, see Sect. 6.4.2.

18.7 Timing of IPR

The timing of the IPR is ideally based on two intraoral features:

(a) The amount of crowding
(b) The degree of contact point displacement

The timing of the IPR can in turn be:

- Left to the AI's default settings
- Specified by the clinician for each individual case
- Generally set by the clinician in the clinical preferences section

It is advisable to always perform IPR on a case-per-case basis. In case of significant crowding, it is also advisable that contact points are rendered more accessible first as premature IPR on rotated teeth can sever the interdental contact areas irreparably. This could result in less-than-ideal contact points at the end of treatment.

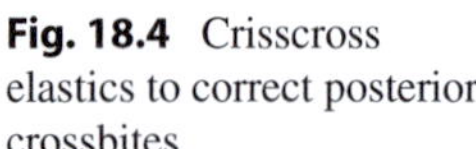

Fig. 18.4 Crisscross elastics to correct posterior crossbites

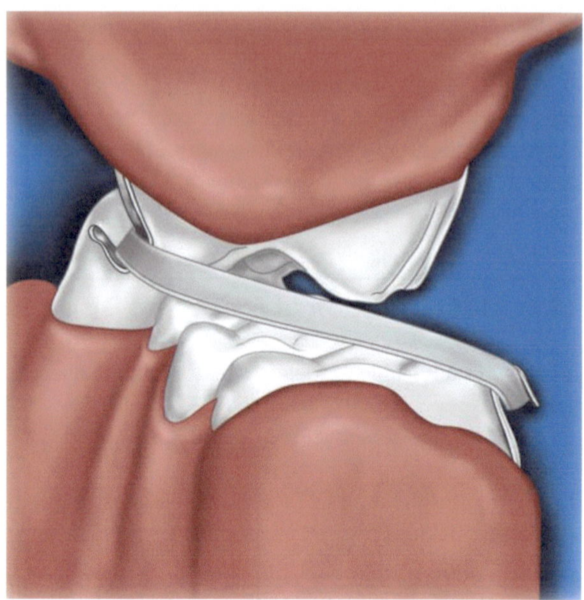

18.8   Posterior Crossbite Correction

Posterior crossbites defined as an abnormal transverse relationship between the buccal segments in the maxillary and mandibular arches leading to the buccal cusps of the maxillary teeth occluding with the central fossae of the mandibular teeth [19]. The prevalence rates have been estimated to be between 8% and 16% but can also be as high as 22% [20, 21]. Correction of posterior crossbites could be challenging to address with aligners only. Relapse is also highly synonymous with posterior crossbite correction with a third of finished cases estimated to undergo unwanted tooth movement [22]. It is thus considered a feature that could repeatedly be the causative factor behind prolonged treatments.

In cases showing very slow no progress or very slow progress in tooth movement especially if lack of tracking is also tangibly visible, the use of inter arch elastics in a crisscross direction may be indicated. Figure 18.4 below shows how these elastics can be placed by the treating clinician.

18.9   Altering the Rate of Staged Correction

Clinicians using clear aligners will have the rate of tooth movement structured on the software's default settings. This in turn will also dictate the individual tooth movements that each tray delivers. Taking Align Technology, Inc., San Jose, Calif, USA aligners, Invisalign®, the automatic settings for each tray include the following tooth movement velocities:

- 2° of de-rotation
- 1° of incisor torque
- 0.25 mm of distalisation

Attempts at increasing the above-mentioned rate of tooth movements will invariably result in decreased accuracy rates. Past studies have estimated that increasing de-rotations beyond 15° resulted in accuracy rates decline between 46% and 52% [11, 23]. The velocity of tooth movement also has a considerable impact on accuracy with rates falling by almost half, scientifically measured as a 44.5% reduction [11].

This highlights the importance of recognising challenging movements and altering the velocity or amount of correction per aligner. A reduction in the velocity and magnitude of tooth movement will ensure that accuracy rates do not decrease significantly and in addition decrease the possibility of tracking issues.

18.10 Careful Selection Between Precision Hooks and Cut-Outs, Their Inclusion and Location

This section deals specifically with precision hooks and cut-outs and aims to deliver two clinical tips which can be useful in the planning stages of a case submitted for clear aligner treatment.

Clinical Tip 1

A very useful clinical tip for a clinician using clear aligner technique is to always allow the software to place the optimised attachments of choice onto the teeth without restriction. This means that the request on the prescription for precision hooks or cut-outs is not submitted at the first ClinCheck® stage or delayed at least. This will allow the clinician to visualise all the necessary multi-planar optimised attachments needed for the planned tooth movement. The possibility of inclusion of the precision hooks or cut-outs should be planned secondary to this.

Clinical Tip 2

The choice between the placement of precision hooks and button cut-outs should be given thorough consideration.

Indication: A-P modification for Class II or Class III malocclusions

Default Software Settings for Precision hooks: Upper canines for class II inter arch elastics and lower canines for class III inter arch elastics.

Default Software Settings for Button Cut-outs: Lower first molars for class II inter arch elastics and upper first molars for class III.

The location of both precision hooks and button cut-outs can be altered on the ClinCheck® Pro 6 by the user.

The factors that should be decisive in choosing the position of the cut-outs are the following:

1. The amount of horizontal vector needed for the sagittal correction.

   In order to decrease the vertical effects of the inter arch elastics and to increase the A-P correction, the cut-outs can be placed on the lower second molars and the upper second molars for class II and class III inter arch elastics, respectively.
2. The number of inter arch elastics intended to be used.

   If more than one elastic band is planned, the precision hooks can be placed on upper and lower first premolars for class II and class III inter arch elastics, respectively. Inversely, the buttons can be placed on the lower second molars and lower first premolars for class II and class III cases, respectively.

The factors that should be decisive in choosing whether precision hooks or button cut-outs are used are given as follows:

1. The degree of torque loss or torque gain needed to the labial segment. The impact on upper and lower labial segment torque is more impactful when a precision hook is used. A button cut-out would provide more isolated tooth movement.
2. The amount of relative extrusion needed to the upper labial segment. Relative extrusion or intrusion is brought about by collective movement of the upper and/ or lower incisors, and therefore it is best accomplished with precision hooks rather than button cut-outs.
3. The degree of individual tooth extrusion needed. Although extrusive movements are difficult to achieve, one way of accomplishing this movement efficiently is to place a button cut-out on the tooth that needs extrusion. This is usually the canines or first premolars or first molars.
4. The amount of distal crown tipping needed. Button cut-outs are much more effective at distal crown tipping than precision hooks especially if these are set advantageously for this movement.
5. The amount of de-rotation needed. Button cut-outs are much more effective at de-rotating canines, premolars and molars depending on the site of placement for the buttons.

References

1. Lima BP, Maio Pinzan-Vercelino CR, Dias LS, Bramante FS, De Jesus Tavarez RR. Correlation between the rotation of the first molars and the severity of class II division 1 malocclusion. Sci World J. 2015;2015:261485.
2. Dahlquist A, Gebauer U, Ingervall B. The effect of a transpalatal arch for the correction of first molar rotation. Eur J Orthod. 1996;18(3):257–67.
3. Vigano CO, da Rocha VE, Junior LRM, Paranhos LR, Ramos AL. Rotation of the upper first molar in class I, II, and III patients. Eur J Dent. 2016;10(1):59–63.
4. Yamunadevi A, Pratibha R, Rajmohan M, Mahendraperumal S, Ganapathy N, Srivandhana R. First molars in permanent dentition and their malformations in various pathologies: a review. J Pharm Bioallied Sci. 2021;13(Suppl 1):S23–30.

5. Bishara SE, Hoppens BJ, Jakobsen JR, Kohout FJ. Changes in the molar relationship between the deciduous and permanent dentitions: a longitudinal study. Am J Orthod Dentofacial Orthop. 1988;93(1):19–28.

6. Lamons FF, Holmes CW III. The problem of the rotated maxillary first permanent molar. Am J Orthod. 1961;47(2):246–72.

7. Braun S, Kusnoto B, Evans CA. The effect of maxillary first molar derotation on arch length. Am J Orthod Dentofacial Orthop. 1997;112(5):538–44.

8. Giuntini V, Baccetti T, Defraia E, Cozza P, Franchi L. Mesial rotation of upper first molars in class II division 1 malocclusion in the mixed dentition: a controlled blind study. Prog Orthod. 2011;12(2):107–13.

9. Zachrisson BU. Important aspects of long-term stability. J Clin Orthod. 1997;31(9):562–83.

10. Ravera S, Castroflorio T, Garino F, Daher S, Cugliari G, Deregibus A. Maxillary molar distalization with aligners in adult patients: a multicenter retrospective study. Prog Orthod. 2016;17:12.

11. Simon M, Keilig L, Schwarze J, Jung BA, Bourauel C. Treatment outcome and efficacy of an aligner technique—regarding incisor torque, premolar derotation and molar distalization. BMC Oral Health. 2014;14:68.

12. Garino F, Castroflorio T, Daher S, Ravera S, Rossini G, Cugliari G, et al. Effectiveness of composite attachments in controlling upper-molar movement with aligners. J Clin Orthod. 2016;50(6):341–7.

13. Morales-Burruezo I, Gandia-Franco JL, Cobo J, Vela-Hernandez A, Bellot-Arcis C. Arch expansion with the Invisalign system: efficacy and predictability. PLoS One. 2020;15(12):e0242979.

14. Houle JP, Piedade L, Todescan R Jr, Pinheiro FH. The predictability of transverse changes with Invisalign. Angle Orthod. 2017;87(1):19–24.

15. Maree A, Kerr B, Weir T, Freer E. Clinical expression of programmed rotation and uprighting of bilateral winged maxillary central incisors with the Invisalign appliance: a retrospective study. Am J Orthod Dentofacial Orthop. 2022;161(1):74–83.

16. Haouili N, Kravitz ND, Vaid NR, Ferguson DJ, Makki L. Has Invisalign improved? A prospective follow-up study on the efficacy of tooth movement with Invisalign. Am J Orthod Dentofacial Orthop. 2020;158(3):420–5.

17. Gaddam R, Freer E, Kerr B, Weir T. Reliability of torque expression by the invisalign appliance: a retrospective study. Aust Orthod J. 2021;37(1):3–13.

18. Blundell HLD, Weir TD, Kerr BD, Freer ED. Predictability of overbite control with the Invisalign appliance. Am J Orthod Dentofacial Orthop. 2021;160(5):725–31.

19. Macena MC, Katz CR, Rosenblatt A. Prevalence of a posterior crossbite and sucking habits in Brazilian children aged 18-59 months. Eur J Orthod. 2009;31(4):357–61.

20. Kisling E. Occlusal interferences in the primary dentition. ASDC J Dent Child. 1981;48(3):181–91.

21. Lindner A, Modeer T. Relation between sucking habits and dental characteristics in preschool-children with unilateral cross-bite. Scand J Dent Res. 1989;97(3):278–83.

22. Almeida RR, Almeida MR, Oltramari-Navarro PV, Conti AC, Navarro Rde L, Marques HV. Posterior crossbite—treatment and stability. J Appl Oral Sci. 2012;20(2):286–94.

23. Kravitz ND, Kusnoto B, BeGole E, Obrez A, Agran B. How well does Invisalign work? A prospective clinical study evaluating the efficacy of tooth movement with Invisalign. Am J Orthod Dentofacial Orthop. 2009;135(1):27–35.

Part IV

Technological Apps to Aid Aligner Therapy

Aligner-Related Apps

19

19.1   Introduction

This chapter focuses on the use and benefits of computer apps and more specifically with orthodontic-related apps where aligners are the appliance of choice. The Covid-19 pandemic and temporary closure of all outlets in the western world has led to a more positive outlook to remote use of apps to facilitate the progress of treatment.

Align Technology, Inc., has developed its own apps for Invisalign®; however, other independent companies have developed their own apps for one or a combination of the domains mentioned above. The apps and their descriptions included in this chapter is not meant to be a finite matter. Contrarily, this aspect of technology will remain very fluid due to the ongoing market influences on these technologies and new apps will be continuously developed and launched.

Align Technology, Inc., provides an online portal for registered users of the system. Online support is available in the form of marketing, educational, and smile projection tools. These are listed below:

Practice marketing toolkit: This sub-section of the portal provides the users with marketing tools that would assist them with disseminating information to clients that are looking at being provided with aligner treatment.

eLearning Platform: This aspect of the portal will provide the user with ten modules for in-depth content about the use of the system to increase the users' knowledge and help them gain familiarisation with the products.

SmileView in-practice tool: This tool offers prospective Invisalign® patients the possibility of viewing the potential post-treatment smile. The end result can be used to set the requirements of the patients in terms of end results.

S. Abela, *Aligner Systems in Invisible Orthodontics*,
https://doi.org/10.1007/978-3-031-49204-4_19

19.2   Invisalign Photo Uploader

Url: https://apps.apple.com/gb/app/invisalign-photo-uploader/id1159148906
    Developer: Align Technology, Inc.,
    Domain: Record keeping
    Description:
Designed mainly for tablet use, the app is also available on iPhones. It is restricted to Invisalign® users only and allows the same users to upload the patient photos swiftly from the portable device which are then made available on the online platform. It provides templates for the photos to be taken in a standardised format and is also able to use AI to accept or reject the quality of the photos submitted.

19.3   Invisalign Pro Consultation App

Url: https://apps.apple.com/gb/app/invisalign-pro-consultation/id1091017497
    Developer; Align Technology, Inc., California, US
    Domain: Educational
    Description:
This app, called Invisalign Pro Consultation, is available on the doctor's site. It is tablet-based, and it is educational in nature. It allows Invisalign® providers to demonstrate the system highlighting the ease of use and all the steps involved. The app also contains stored images, general information and other relevant material in addition to any material uploaded by the user.

Typically, a user might use this app to show the options of treatment including the different levels of Invisalign®, the ClinCheck Pro®, and to show treated cases to show the range of malocclusions that can be treated with aligners. These are classified based on the type of malocclusion so that a prospective patient can identify more with the type of treatment they might need.

19.4   My Invisalign™ App

Url: https://apps.apple.com/gb/app/my-invisalign/id1505554652
    Developer: Align Technology, Inc., California, US
    Domain: Reminders, Progress Monitoring
    Description:
This app allows users to view their 3D simulation readily by accessing it on their phones. The app, mainly developed for iPhones and Apple Watch, is useable before and during treatment. It acts as a reminder for all future appointments sending notifications when follow-up appointments are due. It has a custom timer as a feature to track the number of hours of aligner wear. The user is also able to use the app to share the obtained progress with third party users.

19.5 Other Available Apps

1. TrayMinder®
   Url: https://apps.apple.com/us/app/trayminder-invisalign-tracker/
   id1320684802
   Developer: TrayMinder LLC
   Domain: Reminder app
   Other Products/Related Features: TEETH SElfie™
   Description:
   TrayMinder® app is available on iPhone and Apple Watch and allows the user
   to track the wear time of their aligners. This app is compatible with all aligners
   and is not limited to a single make. The number of hours is tracked on a daily
   basis with a feature called the Timer. Reminders are automatically sent when the
   time is due to change to the next aligner with the in-built feature called the
   Calendar.
   TEETH SElfie™, a feature of this app, allows the user to take selfies to sub-
   stantiate the changes occurring with each aligner change enabling the user to
   really track the tooth movements. The original photos and the progress photos
   would also be available for complete tracking of the changes. These notifications
   are also available on Apple Watch users.

2. Dental Monitoring (DM)
   Url: https://dental-monitoring.com/for-patients/#GetPatientApp
   Developer: Dental Monitoring
   Domain: Remote Monitoring
   Other Products/Apps: SmileMate and 360° Solution
   Description:

Dental Monitoring

Dental Monitoring® (DM) by Dental Monitoring Co., Paris, France is a form
of tele-medicine or tele-orthodontics if there is such a terminology. This involves
aligner progress monitoring from a distance, precluding the need of a patient to
attend the dental surgery. This distant monitoring with the use of an app, helps
aligner treatment surpass other types of treatment in regard to efficiency and
decreased chair-side time. In-built AI within the app enables the software to
detect ongoing deficiencies such as lack of tracking, loss of attachments and
need to re-take intraoral scans or dental impressions. Although this technology
does not eliminate visits to the practice to meet face to face with the treating
clinician, it enables a reduction of visits. The patient benefits from less travelling
and feels more in control of their progress.

The initial set-up would require the patient to download the DM app on their
mobile, whilst the treating clinician would provide support to upload the first
records. This allows the patient to gain familiarity. Any progress records can be
taken at the patients' own convenience and uploaded directly on the app.

SmileMate

SmileMate is a software providing an online assessment through an AI. This is a form of diagnostic tool that assists treating clinicians understand a prospective new patient's needs and type of malocclusion that needs addressing.

360° Solution

This is the name given by DM representing the encompassing of all the digital solutions on offer by the company.

360° Solution offers the initial assessment software package, digital simulation of the projected end result and the remote monitoring software.

3. Aligner Consult

   Url: https://apps.apple.com/se/app/aligner-consult/id1258919849

   Developer: Brightsquid Dental Ltd., Calgary, Alberta, Canada

   Domain: Diagnostics

   Other Products/Features: Secure-Mail

   Description:

   Brightsquid Secure Communications Corp. doesn't deliver the above app only. It aims to reconfigure healthcare delivery involving numerous specialists and professionals. This is facilitated by an open forum that allows sharing of medical information between the professionals involved in the healthcare of an individual. This is secure and avoids delays between correspondences.

   With regard to the orthodontic app similarly allows capture of photos and information for easy access by the company's aligners consultants.

   The app is compatible with Apple iPhones, iPad and MacBook laptops.

4. Invisalign Practice App

   Url: https://apps.apple.com/us/app/invisalign-practice-app/id1570887123?platform=iphone

   Developer: Align Technology, Inc., California, US

   Domain: Diagnostics, Reminder

   Description:

   This app is reserved for Invisalign-registered users. Available on iPad, iPhone and MacBook laptops, it allows digitisation of patient records and it automatically syncs with the online portal.

   It is diagnostic verifying suitability for treatment with Invisalign Go, whilst it also remotely monitors progress.

   The virtual appointment feature allows the introduction of the prospective patient with the treating clinician.

5. Aligner Smile Tracker

   Url: https://apps.apple.com/us/app/aligner-smile-tracker/id1535341862

   Developer: © Pocketpixels 2021

   Seller: Dean Martin

   Other Related Products: Clearaligner Smartortho App

   Domain: Diagnostics, Reminders

   Description:

Aligner Smile Tracker

This app designed to be used on iPhones mainly, allows tracking of the need to change aligners and when the day is due for the next aligner to be changed.

It incorporates a calendar to set up dates for aligner changes, a gallery to place all photos, and a progress video section that builds footage based on the photos taken and uploaded.

The reminder feature of the app is dual use; it is able to remind the patient when to change the aligner but also sets a reminder when the number of hours the aligners are not in use has been exceeded to increase compliance.

Clearaligner Smartortho App

Principally, a diagnostic app allowing uploading of patients' photos to certify suitability for treatment using aligners.

6. TrayTime

    Url: https://apps.apple.com/gb/app/traytime/id1250940516
    Developer: Pocketglow LLC
    Domain: Reminders
    Description:

    TrayTime is an app restricted to Invisalign® users with the aim of tracking the number of hours of usage and non-usage of each tray. The app is also compatible with Apple Watch and aims to increase patient compliance. Features of the app allows a timer indicating "On" when the tray is being used and "Off" when the aligner is not being used. The default number of hours is 22 h a day as recommended by the manufacturer.

7. Aligner Global Community

    Url: https://apps.apple.com/us/app/id1592346603
    Seller: Aligner Consultancy Limited
    Domain: Educational/Informative
    Description:

    This app developed by the Aligner Global Community (AGC) aims to collate aligner users. It provides details for courses, provides advice and mentoring for beginners and the platform introduces users to each other.

8. RemindAlign

    Url: https://apps.apple.com/gb/app/remindalign/id1192710002
    Developer: HHPage Inc.
    Domain: Reminder
    Description:

    Mainly available for iPad and iPhone use, this app acts as a reminder on when the aligners need to be changed. Alerts are sent depending on the settings chosen.

9. StrojCHECK®

    Url: https://apps.apple.com/fj/app/strojcheck/id1540962621
    Developer: 3Dent medical s. r. o., Bratislava, Slovakia
    Domain: Reminder
    Description:

    This app which is compatible with MacBooks, iPhones and iPads is developed in Bratislava. It assists aligner users to maintain usage for the required number of hours.

Part V

Evidence-Based Aligner Therapy

Scientific Evidence of Aligner Treatment   20

20.1   Introduction

The last few years have witnessed the introduction and a widespread uptake of computer-aided design (CAD) and computer-aided manufacturing (CAM) technologies. This in turn has given easier access to aligners and their use as a mainstream technique in orthodontics and dentistry in general.

This trend can also be reflected in the amount of scientific evidence being produced in this area. The greatest contributions as illustrated in Fig. 20.1 below, obtained from PubMed, part of PubMed Central®, a collection of biomedical and life science journals at the National Library of Medicine (NLM) at the United States National Institute of Health (NIH), shows an upward trend of such work being produced in the last few years. The diagram illustrates scientific work published from 1966 with evidence that the highest concentration is found in the past two decades.

On closer inspection with a much-focused search, no scientific data is present before 2003. Two of the first studies published investigated the precision of Align Technology, Inc., three-dimensional computer-based prediction methodologies [1, 2]. This indicates that most of the studies available are from this date onwards, which to date, means a span of approximately 20 years.

With such an uptake in treatment especially in adults, both specialists and general dental practitioners are increasingly recurring to using this technique. In the past decade, there has also been a surge in systematic reviews (SRs) and meta-analyses (MAs), considered to be the highest level of evidence possible, mostly comparing aligners with the gold standard; fixed appliances. Chronologically, Rossini et al. provided one of the first systematic reviews focusing on the patients' periodontal health during aligner therapy, whilst the second systematic review focused on the efficacy of tooth movement [3, 4]. Other SRs followed in 2017 by Elhaddaoui et al. and Zheng et al. and in 2018 by Aldeeri et al., Jiang et al. Lu et al. and Papadimitriou et al. [5, 6–10] In 2019 contributions followed by Galan-Lopez et al., Ke et al. and Fang et al. [11–13]

© The Author(s), under exclusive license to Springer Nature Switzerland AG 2024   159
S. Abela, *Aligner Systems in Invisible Orthodontics*,
https://doi.org/10.1007/978-3-031-49204-4_20

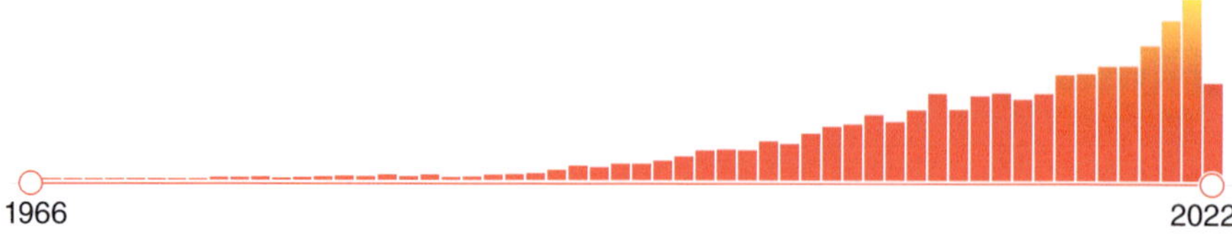

Fig. 20.1 A PubMed search on "clear aligners" showing the upward trend in producing evidence-based data on this technique mostly concentrated in the last few years

The very latest SRs available include those of Robertson et al., Cardoso et al., Ghandi et al., Zhang et al., Oikonomou et al., Ali Baeshen et al., Ben Gassem et al., Nucera et al., Yassir et al., Bakdach et al., Mheissen et al. and Al-Zainal et al. [14, 15, 16, 17, 18–25]

20.2   Changes in Chemical and Mechanical Properties of Aligners During Use

By simply considering the materials constituting most aligners on the market, it is very acceptable to assume a degree of deterioration from intraoral use. The original state of the aligner is not maintained over time, and this could contribute from a downward shift in the aligners' performance from its originally intended purpose [26]. This has been investigated in multiple studies with some of the deteriorations observed included, surface cracks, abrasion defects, calcification, adsorption and ion exchange amongst others [27, 28].

The thermoforming process involved in the production of aligners has permanent and lasting effects on the physical and mechanical properties of the aligner material used [29]. This is also applicable to SmartTrack's LD30. Despite being the most commonly used material given the position of Invisalign® as the market leader, both mechanical and chemical changes are observed to the surface morphology which could in turn deliver sub-optimal clinical results [16]. In a study available in the literature, various materials were selected however only LD30 that met the stipulated inclusion criteria, it still exhibited distortion of surface topology and ions exchange was observed with intraoral usage. Indentation modulus (EIT) and Martens hardness (HM) were used as markers as they represent force delivery and wear resistance, respectively.

In another prospective clinical study, the physical deterioration of clear aligners over 10 days of intraoral use was investigated. The rationale for the investigative time was purely due to the tendency of in vivo time that patients tend to wear the aligners for. The thickness of the aligner material in this study was studied using different occlusal points on a 3D model. Two types of aligners were used: one passive maxillary aligner and one active maxillary aligner. None of the aligners, passive or active showed clinically significant physical changes [30].

20.3 Periodontal Health During Aligner Treatment

The iatrogenic effects of orthodontic treatment are well-known, have been well researched and reported in the literature too. Complications to the periodontal status is one of the most frequently observed complications together with root resorption [31]. Historically, the pathophysiological process involved the build-up of higher levels of plaque biofilm post-placement of fixed appliances. The plaque build-up, the main aetiological factor in a periodontal status downgrade, could if not addressed further accumulate and invade the sub-gingival pockets, leading to further deterioration of the periodontal status [32]. The manifestation of this phenomenon would lead to gingivitis, gingival bleeding, gingival hyperplasia, increased periodontal pocket depths and in case of demineralisation, white spot lesions [33]. In addition, to the above changes, findings from previously published studies include changes to the bacterial composition and increased retention [34, 35].

The introduction of clear aligners has eliminated the adhesion aspect of fixed appliances and the possibility of removing the appliances for better hygiene has resulted in better periodontal health. In a study evaluating the real-time accumulation and presence of microbiological biofilms over a 3-month period using polymerase chain reaction (PCR) has shown superior periodontal health status amongst patients receiving Invisalign® treatment in contrast to patients receiving fixed appliance therapy [31].

A systematic review carried out in 2015 by Rossini et al. included five prospective studies, of which 1 was a randomised controlled trial [3]. The evidence level being judged as moderate, with the recommendation of interpreting the conclusions of the study with caution due to inaccuracies and biases found in the studies included. A meta-analysis could not be included due a high degree of heterogeneity. The authors have placed great emphasis on the patients' oral hygiene regimes as a lack of the latter is the main causative factor for the maintenance of the periodontal status. In four out of five of the studies included the Plaque Index (PI) was significantly lower in patients with clear aligners than those receiving fixed appliance therapy. Other periodontal indices: Gingival Index (GI), Papillary Bleeding Index (PBI), Bleeding on Probing (BoP) and Periodontal Pocket Depth (PPD) were also reported better in patients receiving aligner therapy in contrast to treatment with fixed appliances.

In a different study, based in South Korea, the effects of fixed appliances (FA) and clear aligners (CA) were explored in patients with periodontitis. All the patients selected for the study after receiving the necessary oral hygiene instructions were examined and the periodontal indices, used as clinical parameters were registered. In both groups, all patients showed an improvement in hygiene levels and no significant differences were noted in PI and GI [36].

In a separate three-arm parallel-group prospective randomised clinical trial by Chhibber et al., completed in 2017, a comparison of the long-term and short-term effects of clear aligners with self-ligated brackets and conventional fixed appliances on patients' oral hygiene. Three timelines for measurement of the periodontal indices were used: at the start of treatment, 9 months and 18 months into treatment. No significant differences in oral hygiene were noticed between the three different types of appliances in the long term. In the short term, patients with clear aligners had better GI and PBI scores than those with FA. Not enough evidence was found to direct a clinician to choose one type of appliance from another. Although CAs are broadly associated with better periodontal prospects [37], the coverage of the aligners over the hard and soft tissue prevents the natural flushing of the oral cavity with saliva. This could result in a higher accumulation of plaque biofilm and carious lesions alike [38].

In a meta-analysis by Jiang et al. in 2018, the study's findings favoured CAs over FAs for periodontal health during active treatment [8].

In cases that need expansion as part of the treatment, a study using Invisalign® has shown that there is no deterioration in periodontal health status nor in the buccal bone in the first and premolar regions. The findings were recorded for the first 12 months of treatment and used both clinical and tomographic images for the interpretation of the data [39]. This study was sponsored by Align tech which could be considered as a bias.

The most recent systematic review and meta-analysis on the impact of CAs and FAs on oral health was published in 2021. Accepting the limitations of the studies included with a high level of heterogeneity and bias, short-term benefits of oral hygiene with patients receiving CAs treatment in the short term was recognised.

20.4   Effect of the Type of Attachment on Aligner Treatment

Various studies have been carried out researching the benefits of attachments and their contribution towards treatment outcomes.

The attachments can be used for improved aligner retention or to enhance tooth movement. One of the first studies with the aim of investigating this was in 2015 by Day et al. carried out on stone casts using ellipsoid, rectangular and no attachments with the latter serving as a control [40]. Although the findings of this study cannot be extrapolated to a clinical setting directly, the authors have shown that bevelled attachments were superior at improving the retention of aligners in comparison to having ellipsoid or no attachments at all.

In 2019, Mantovani et al. provided a study using Scanning Electron Microscopy (SEM) analysing the fit of three different aligners; Invisalign by Align Technology, Santa Clara, CA, USA, CA Clear Aligner by Scheu-Dental, Iserlohn, Germany and F22 by Sweden & Martina, Due Carrare, Italy over the anchorage attachments. The study also analysed the effect of using two different types of resin used to build attachments on aligner fitting. All three types of aligners had similar performances with the attachments whilst conventional composite performed better than flowable composite.

20.5 Comparison Between Treatment with Fixed Appliances and Aligners

Numerous studies have now been carried out comparing the two types of systems which provide most of the orthodontic treatments; fixed appliances (FA) and clear aligners (CA).

20.5.1 Efficiency of Aligner Treatment

A systematic review and meta-analysis analysing the effectiveness and efficiency of CAs was first carried out in 2017. Overall strong evidence was found to be lacking however for mild to moderate cases treated with CAs, chair-side time and treatment duration seemed to be superior over FA cases [5].

In another systematic review carried out a year later in 2018, the accuracy of tooth movement with Invisalign® was analysed for each of the studies available. In total, two studies with high quality evidence were included together with 7 with moderate level of evidence and 5 with low evidence [12]. In this study, the authors recognised that the intercanine and intermolar widths are more often than not altered during treatment. This is also the case with incisor proclination in the presence of crowding. In addition, the findings included that the least predictable tooth movements are de-rotations and tooth movements in the vertical dimension such as intrusion and extrusion. This is in line with other studies for both de-rotations [41] and vertical movements [42]. Additional techniques for the former type of movement are recommended when the correction exceeds 15° of de-rotation movement. For the latter type of movement, attachments are crucial for the success of any vertical movement.

Other recommendations include personalisation of the frequency of change of aligners rather than a generalised approach with a weekly change for each stage of aligners. FAs remain superior to CAs with regard to precision and control of tooth movement. This is also in line with the findings of other studies; [43] hence, the additional recommendation to overcorrect the movements on the ClinCheck Pro® software as it is more likely that the end result is more similar to the predicted one. The effects of the appliance on root movements are limited.

In a slight contradiction to the above findings, a systematic review by Kassam et al. found that although CA can be successful at treating class I malocclusions involving extractions, the treatment time is not shorter than conventional FAs. Similar to the other authors' findings treatment with CAs were inferior at stability postoperatively and obtaining successful final occlusal outcomes [44].

In a further overview of systematic reviews aimed at further distinguishing the benefits of using FAs or CAs, the authors concluded that aligners are beneficial to the treatment and could be considered as an effective treatment alternative however less so for more complex cases [25].

Accuracy of the tooth movement prediction was published following a prospective study [45]. The authors of this study concluded that the 15th stage of the CA is a pivotal stage to ascertain accuracy of real-life tooth movement in comparison to the digital prediction.

20.5.2 Quantification of Efficiency of Aligner Treatment

One of the initial studies looking at quantifying the amount of tooth movements was reported by Joffe et al. [46] The articles entitled "Early Experiences" reflects the initial stages of Invisalign's presence in the market; however, the quantification assists the clinician with assessing the feasibility of using CAs to address specific type of malocclusions. The authors suggested that the selection criteria should exclude malocclusions with the following occlusal features:

- Spacing and/or crowding of more than 5 mm
- Skeletal antero-posterior discrepancies of greater than 2 mm
- Interocclusal discrepancies
- De-rotational movement of greater than 20°
- Open bites (anterior or posterior)
- Extrusive movements
- Crown tipping of greater than 45°
- Short clinical crowns
- Hypodontia

Further attempts at quantification of the tooth movement accuracy has been measured at 47.1% [47]. The authors of the same study measured extrusive movement prediction at 29.6%, that is the clinical outcome was only one third of the planned movement. Precision of extrusive movements of maxillary incisors and mandibular incisors were 18.3% and 24.5%, respectively. Mesio-distal tipping of mandibular canines was 26.9%. De-rotational correction was worst for upper lateral incisors followed by canines. The most predictable movement was lingual constriction at 47.1%. Replication of the digital prediction of buccal crown tipping for incisors was also poor.

The most predictable movement was distalisation of buccal segments which was high at 88%. Translation of movement in a buccopalatal inclination in the buccal segments was also successful but less so in the labial segments.

Numerical quantification of digital to clinical realisation was shown in another study by Simon et al. The overall efficacy was 59% with a lower figure for upper incisor toque with the least predictable movement being de-rotations with an accuracy figure of 40%. Distalisation was also shown to be the most predictable movement at 87% [41].

A study using the American Board of Orthodontists (ABO) objective grading system (OGS) showed similar improvements with both types of appliances [43] however in a separate retrospective study using OGS, Invisalign scored much less than FAs. Further limitations were highlighted in other studies with clear superiority of FAs over CAs in the following aspects:

- Effectiveness of treatment [48]
- Occlusal outcomes [49, 50]
- Transverse correction [51]
- Postoperative stability [52]
- Vertical finishing with FAs allowing extrusive movements of up to 0.5 mm [12, 13]
- Postoperative interdigitation in the buccal segments [13]
- Root control and torque expression [41, 49]
- Need of compliance [53]
- Proclination of teeth [3]

The CAs were superior in maintaining the original inclination of teeth and less able to procline the labial segments which could be advantageous in patients with a very thin gingival biotype or those with existing recession defects. This is also beneficial in camouflage cases with the aim of maintaining the inclination of the compensated labial segments in either arch. The CAs were also more efficient as mentioned above in a meta-analysis carried out by Zheng et al. with regard to chairside time and treatment duration. The latter however applies to non-extraction cases as those requiring extractions had longer treatment durations by up to 44% [43]. This was mostly applicable to cases with premolar extractions.

In another study further supporting CA as a mainstream treatment, the authors conducted a prospective study. The accuracy of tooth movement was the highest recorded in the literature. The overall accuracy was 86% with a range of 96% for maxillary central incisors to 70.4% for mandibular first premolars [54].

20.5.3 Impact of Aligner Treatment on the Smile Outcome

The outcome that is fundamentally most important to the patient is the change in smile aesthetics. In a case-control study, smile outcomes between FAs and CAs were directly compared [55].

This study was a retrospective study based on records which were available on a database. Fifteen variables were used as parameters to measure the smile outcome. No significant differences in postoperative scores were highlighted between the two modalities; however, FAs were shown to be more effective at most variables that determine post-treatment smiles outcome. CAs represented in this study by Invisalign® were superior in improving the maxillary position and inclination.

20.5.4 Radiological Assessment of the Effect of Aligners on the Treatment Outcome

A radiologically based study specifically aimed at evaluating the radiological impact of aligner treatment on tooth movement was successfully carried out using conebeam computed tomography (CBCT). The study was a retrospective study based on

69 patients that underwent CA treatment with Invisalign®. Pre- and post-treatment CBCTs were superimposed over the ClinCheck prediction [56].

The overall efficacy of Invisalign® for all incisor movements in the sagittal plane was 55.58%. The highest accuracy, reflecting the removable nature of the appliance was achieved during pure tipping with the prediction levels reaching 72.48%. The second accurate movement was controlled tipping at 65.24% and translation with levels reaching 49.50%. The lowest accuracy movement was torque with prediction levels decreasing to almost one third of the digital simulation at 35.21%. Inter arch differences were only observed for translation movements of the maxillary incisors being less effective in a significant way when compared to the mandibular incisors. In an antero-posterior dimension, labial tooth movements were more predictable than movements in a lingual direction. In the same direction, the maxillary incisors showed less predictable movement than lower incisors; 51.03% versus 60.01% for mandibular incisors. With regard to the efficacy of movement the lower incisors also scored higher; 56.16% versus 69.52% for the mandibular incisors. Overall, the results highlighted poor lingual root movement and buccal root movement for upper incisors was more difficult to achieve than for lower incisors.

Another CBCT-based study looking at anterior intrusion with Invisalign® aligners in 2021 showed that the efficacy of intrusion was 51.9%. The highest precision figure was obtained from intrusive moments of maxillary lateral incisors with an efficacy of 58.12%. The least accurate figure was obtained from infusion of mandibular incisors at 44.71%. In the maxilla, the central incisors demonstrated a figure of 51.83% whilst maxillary canines scored 48.95%. Mandibular canines scored slightly more at 52.34%. The intrusive value in millimetres was measured at less than 1 mm; 0.9 mms [57]. This is in line with the above-referenced study by Kravitz et al. where the sum of intrusive movement was 0.72 mm [47].

In a cephalometric-based study, the changes in molar position in a vertical dimension was assessed and compared in both FA and CA treatment [58]. This study although a retrospective study provided an inferior outcome for vertical molar control with CAs when compared to FAs.

Using CBCTs and specifically looking at the adequacy of CA to distalise buccal segments in the mandibular arch, Wu et al. analysed the movements of the first and second molars [59]. The efficiency of movement was better for mandibular second molars for both crowns and roots. The first molar crown and root efficacy was 71% and 47% in contrast to crown and root movement for second molars which was better at 74% and 49%. The distalisation movement was associated with intrusion, buccal and distal tipping. There were no differences between male and female participants in the study.

20.6   Aligner Treatment Effects on Root Resorption

External apical root resorption (EARR) is a common iatrogenic effect of orthodontic treatment. EARR is usually a phenomenon due to biological and mechanical factors. Although biological factors can't be manipulated, mechanical factors such as degree of force, duration of force, amount of tooth movement and type of appliance can be altered to decrease the occurrence. Multiple studies have also been carried out to distinguish any increased risk of having an increased rate of EARR depending on the type of appliance used. FAs or CAs have been compared with this regard.

In a retrospective study, using radiographical analyses of root lengths, CAs were shown to induce less EARR than FA [60]. The findings in a pilot study using a radiographical assessment and comparing self-ligating fixed appliances and Invisalign® has also shown similar findings [61].

In a systematic review aiming at providing further evidence of EARR with FA or CA using 3D measurements could only include two studies with high-level evidence. The conclusions included a low-risk association with CA [7].

An additional systematic review looking at EARR investigating the incidence of EARR in patients receiving FA and CAs has also shown a decreased risk [11]. Al-Zainal et al. have also shown that although CAs do not eliminate the risk of EARR, there is a significantly reduced risk when compared to the occurrence with FAs [18].

A study based in the United States and published in the *European Journal of Orthodontics* have also found non-significant differences between pre-adjusted edgewise appliances and CA with regard to the occurrence of EARR. The only significant difference was found in EARR affecting the upper right lateral incisors [62].

A study using CBCTs to further distinguish any significant clinical differences between FAs and CAs also concluded that EARR is less when CAs are used [63]. CBCTs were also used by Liu et al. to investigate the prevalence of EARR during CA treatment and identify any risk factors that could exacerbate it [64]. The authors have found only mild to moderate level of EARR. The risk factors included sagittal changes in root position, extraction cases, tooth type and tooth movements in the vertical dimension predominantly extrusion and intrusion.

In a different study, the same aspects as the above studies were investigated through a randomised clinical trial in the first 6 months of treatment [65]. For both types of appliances, the EARR in the first 6 months of treatment was not significant, and there were no differences reported between the two types of appliances.

20.7 Changes in Bacterial Counts and Groups

The iatrogenic effects of orthodontic treatment are both well-known and well researched. FAs are also a well-known causative factor for enamel demineralisation by decreasing the ability to clean the tooth surfaces and by altering the oral microflora which is a consequence of an increase in plaque scores. These increased plaque scores invariably lead to an increase in the bacterial count of *Streptococcus mutans (S. mutans)*, one of the main bacterial species leading to the development of new or recurrent carious lesions, amongst others [66, 67].

CAs in a similar way have raised suspicions of an increased risk of being the cause of an oral microflora alteration favouring increased counts of *S. mutans and*

Lactobacillus species (Lactobacillus ssp.). One of the first prospective cohort studies looking into this was carried out using a prospective cohort of adolescent patients aged 12–18 years. The patients in the cohort were assigned to FAs or CAs followed for 1 month, after which they progressed to having conventional FAs. Although this study had a very limited follow-up period of 1 month and the cohort was not randomised, no significant differences can be found between the two types of appliances in terms of bacterial levels of cariogenic bacteria [68].

In another prospective clinical study with a 6-month follow-up, salivary samples were obtained prior to starting treatment and 6 months into the treatment. No significant differences were found in bacterial counts or in oral health status [69].

In another observational study looking at bacterial counts of Streptococcus and Lactobacilli over the first 6 months of treatment. FAs, CAs and removable positioners (RPs) were used during the study. The FA group had a much higher bacterial count of these two bacterial groups that could in turn lead to a higher risk of dental decay. In this group, the increase observed was 20% in the first 3 months and 40% at 6 months into treatment. This is significantly higher to the increased counts for the CA and RP groups with observed increase of 10 and 13%, respectively [70].

A wide literature review analysing all of the literature available was provided to us by Contaldo et al. in 2021. The article encompasses all the available literature describing the effects of FAs, components of FAs, different types of FA and CAs on the oral microflora composition [71]. The study also highlights the difference in microflora changes in patients with systemic diseases and also highlights the increased count of *Candida spp.* which in turn results in higher incidences of oral candidiasis.

The changes in sub-gingival species was investigated by a team based in Ferrara, Italy [72]. Real-time PCR was used to verify the bacterial counts and a comparison was drawn between these count verifications in FA and CA groups. Different time points were also selected to draw up the counts. The total bacterial count in the former group was much higher and increased progressively throughout treatment up to 6 months which was the total observation period. The bacterial count remained stable in the CA group.

In a comparative study with follow-ups of 12 months between FA and CA groups once more, the Plaque and Gingival Indices were better with the latter group. It was also found that the aligners attract a specific type of microbial communities [73].

20.8 Comparing Outcomes in Orthognathic Surgical Cases

In recent times, aligners have also been considered as an alternative appliance to the conventional fixed appliances. Historically, FAs were considered to be the gold standard in orthognathic surgery cases and FAs were considered to produce the optimal outcomes needed to treat such cases.

The authors, Kankam et al., in 2019 produced one of the first studies investigating the feasibility of using CA in favour of FAs. The authors aimed at verifying the use of CA as an alternative to FA and comparing orthognathic outcomes between the two groups of patients. The conclusion verified that orthognathic surgery was successful even when CAs were used [74].

In a very different study, with a surgery-first approach, CAs were used to assess outcomes based on a case report. The study has managed to show the benefits of having surgery first but also the added benefit of being able to finish the postoperative orthodontic treatment with CAs [75]. From a clinical perspective Lou et al. 2021 provide a detailed clinical description of the sequences to successfully treat patients with orthognathic surgery using clear aligner therapy.

In a case report, Invisalign® was shown to be effective as a treatment for patients receiving orthognathic surgery. In this publication, the case reported a 19-year-old male that was successfully treated with a bimaxillary osteotomy involving a Le Fort I and a bilateral sagittal split osteotomy (BSSO) [76].

20.9 Comparing Pain Experiences of Patients Having Aligner Treatment

Another differentiating characteristic between FA and CA groups is the pain perception during treatment. Various studies have aimed at featuring any differences in pain perceptions between different type of orthodontic systems.

Pain could be considered a subjective response and will vary depending on the type of subjects in the cohort apart from other variables. The recruitment stage of subjects although randomised will not be able to eliminate all the variables.

One such study is the one conducted by Cardoso et al. in 2020 published in the *Progress in Orthodontics* journal [19]. This systematic review involved orthodontic cases of mild complexity and CAs fared better in this area when compared to FA but only in the first 3 months of treatment.

In another systematic review encompassing both randomised and non-randomised trials, patients' perception of pain with CAs were lower than those receiving FA treatment. This finding was only valid for the first few days of treatment. The level of evidence was considered to be low [20].

Other authors have tried investigating this from a more scientific perspective by investigating cytokine levels in the gingival crevicular fluid (GCF) after insertion of clear aligners [77]. Interleukins are signalling proteins that delineate the presence of inflammation. Interleukin 1 can be found in alpha (α) and beta (β) forms, and the latter was used in this study as it is a biomarker for inflammation. Its elevated levels during treatment can in turn infer tissue remodelling which is needed in orthodontic treatment to demonstrate tooth movement. The authors used the lower labial segment as the experimental site and used the upper arch as control which received no treatment. The findings showed increased levels especially in the first 24 h of aligner application which was inferred as a reflection of successful tooth movement.

Pain induction from over activation of the masticatory muscles of mastication as a result of orthodontic treatment has also been investigated [78]. The study's main limitation, although extremely helpful in their findings, was the very short-term follow-up of 3 months. Using surface electromyography (sEMG), the authors established a statistically significant reduction in the sEMG activity of the masseter muscles at mandibular rest position. The authors took further readings at 1 month and 3 months and have shown that the masseter activity returned to normal levels when the patients were into the third month of their treatment. Due to the lack of alteration of muscular activity and lack of pain originating from the muscles of mastication, the authors further suggested that aligners can be indicated for patients with temporomandibular joint dysfunction (TMJD).

20.10 Effect of Aligner Treatment on the Quality of Life

The quality of life (QoL) aspect of a treatment modality is considered to be a very important factor during treatment provision. Oral health-related QoL (OHRQoL) is a measure of high importance to patients as alternative treatment modalities are available and various choices are available. The treatment option that provides the best QoL improvement should be the default choice and the patient together with the clinician should make this decision together after analysing the evidence in favour and against each treatment option. Systematic reviews and individual studies have been carried out to explore this in much further detail.

A systematic review concluded that to date there is limited evidence on the effects of CA therapy on OHRQoL compared to FA treatment. The review provided weak evidence suggesting that patients receiving CA have better masticatory function compared to those receiving FA treatment [14].

In a very interesting study involving a prospective cohort receiving buccal FA, lingual FA and Ca were compared in terms of QoL benefits. The study was survey-based involving 117 patients. The QoL scores were highest in the group receiving CA [79].

Similar positive findings were also highlighted in a study looking at pain perception, anxiety and OHRQoL scored by the selected cohort of 110 patients. The patients were matched as much as possible by the investigators and were assessed via a visual analogue scale for pain perception, state-trait anxiety inventory to assess anxiety levels and oral health impact profile-14 (OHIP-14) to assess OHRQoL scores. CA scored better in all the three areas when compared to FA [80].

In a randomised controlled trial, CA were also compared to FA in terms of improvement of QoL [81]. All the treatments in the study were based on a non-extraction approach and the study as a two-arm parallel randomised controlled trial (RCT). Patients treated with CA fared better and reported higher OHRQoL than those receiving treatment with FA.

A different RCT with a cohort needing an extraction-approach due to severe crowding was also conducted providing information on the effect of needing more complex and lengthy treatment. The follow-up period was established as 1 year and the OHRQoL using OHIP-14 was also as in previous studies. No significant differences were found in terms of psychological discomfort, psychological and social disability between patients receiving FA and CA. Significant differences were found in functional limitation, physical pain and physical disability with the CA group faring better than the FA group [82].

20.11 Effect of Aligner Treatment on Speech

A very important aspect of orthodontic treatment is the perceived effect on speech by the appliances chosen to deliver the treatment. Speech alteration is considered an adverse effect of treatment and limiting its effect is one of the main aims of the treating clinician. The reduction of intraoral space is described as the main causative factor [83].

Different appliances might be associated with varying degrees of speech impairment and in a comparing Hawley and vacuum-formed retainers, the former was associated with a more significant impairment than the latter [84].

In another study, the maximum time needed for patients to adjust their speech to their new Invisalign® trays took 2 weeks [85]. In another study, the effect on speech, mainly the articulation of certain consonants led to a marked impact [86].

In an RCT attempting to distinguish the impact of FA and CA on speech, the authors found that patients with CA had a larger impact on speech at the time of insertion and 3 days after insertion of the CA. Within 30 days the two groups had a similar impact on speech. The authors also included that both type of appliances had a patient-perceived impairment on speech [87].

In a systematic review specifically aimed at analysing speech impairment, patient perceptions on speech impairment was present with clear aligner type of appliances; however, the patients adapted to this within the initial stages of treatment [23].

References

1. Beers AC, Choi W, Pavlovskaia E. Computer-assisted treatment planning and analysis. Orthod Craniofac Res. 2003;6(Suppl 1):117–25.
2. Miller RJ, Kuo E, Choi W. Validation of align technology's treat III digital model superimposition tool and its case application. Orthod Craniofac Res. 2003;6(Suppl 1):143–9.
3. Rossini G, Parrini S, Castroflorio T, Deregibus A, Debernardi CL. Efficacy of clear aligners in controlling orthodontic tooth movement: a systematic review. Angle Orthod. 2015;85(5):881–9.
4. Rossini G, Parrini S, Castroflorio T, Deregibus A, Debernardi CL. Periodontal health during clear aligners treatment: a systematic review. Eur J Orthod. 2015;37(5):539–43.
5. Zheng M, Liu R, Ni Z, Yu Z. Efficiency, effectiveness and treatment stability of clear aligners: a systematic review and meta-analysis. Orthod Craniofac Res. 2017;20(3):127–33.
6. Elhaddaoui R, Qoraich HS, Bahije L, Zaoui F. Orthodontic aligners and root resorption: a systematic review. Int Orthod. 2017;15(1):1–12.
7. Aldeeri A, Alhammad L, Alduham A, Ghassan W, Shafshak S, Fatani E. Association of orthodontic clear aligners with root resorption using three-dimension measurements: a systematic review. J Contemp Dent Pract. 2018;19(12):1558–64.
8. Jiang Q, Li J, Mei L, Du J, Levrini L, Abbate GM, et al. Periodontal health during orthodontic treatment with clear aligners and fixed appliances: a meta-analysis. J Am Dent Assoc. 2018;149(8):712–20 e12.

9. Lu H, Tang H, Zhou T, Kang N. Assessment of the periodontal health status in patients undergoing orthodontic treatment with fixed appliances and Invisalign system: a meta-analysis. Medicine (Baltimore). 2018;97(13):e0248.

10. Papadimitriou A, Mousoulea S, Gkantidis N, Kloukos D. Clinical effectiveness of Invisalign(R) orthodontic treatment: a systematic review. Prog Orthod. 2018;19(1):37.

11. Fang X, Qi R, Liu C. Root resorption in orthodontic treatment with clear aligners: a systematic review and meta-analysis. Orthod Craniofac Res. 2019;22(4):259–69.

12. Galan-Lopez L, Barcia-Gonzalez J, Plasencia E. A systematic review of the accuracy and efficiency of dental movements with Invisalign(R). Korean J Orthod. 2019;49(3):140–9.

13. Ke Y, Zhu Y, Zhu M. A comparison of treatment effectiveness between clear aligner and fixed appliance therapies. BMC Oral Health. 2019;19(1):24.

14. Zhang B, Huang X, Huo S, Zhang C, Zhao S, Cen X, et al. Effect of clear aligners on oral health-related quality of life: a systematic review. Orthod Craniofac Res. 2020;23(4):363–70.

15. Ben Gassem AA. Does clear aligner treatment result in different patient perceptions of treatment process and outcomes compared to conventional/traditional fixed appliance treatment: a literature review. Eur J Dent. 2022;16(2):274–85.

16. Bakdach WMM, Haiba M, Hadad R. Changes in surface morphology, chemical and mechanical properties of clear aligners during intraoral usage: a systematic review and meta-analysis. Int Orthod. 2022;20(1):100610.

17. Robertson L, Kaur H, Fagundes NCF, Romanyk D, Major P, Flores MC. Effectiveness of clear aligner therapy for orthodontic treatment: a systematic review. Orthod Craniofac Res. 2020;23(2):133–42.

18. Al-Zainal MH, Anvery S, Al-Jewair T. Clear aligner therapy may not prevent but may decrease the incidence of external root resorption compared to full fixed appliances. J Evid Based Dent Pract. 2020;20(2):101438.

19. Cardoso PC, Espinosa DG, Mecenas P, Flores-Mir C, Normando D. Pain level between clear aligners and fixed appliances: a systematic review. Prog Orthod. 2020;21(1):3.

20. Mheissen S, Khan H, Aldandan M. Limited evidence on differences between fixed appliances and clear aligners regarding pain level. Evid Based Dent. 2020;21(4):144–5.

21. Ghandi K, Pieri B, Dornhorst A, Hussain S. A comparison of validated methods used to assess impaired awareness of hypoglycaemia in type 1 diabetes: an observational study. Diabetes Ther. 2021;12(1):441–51.

22. Oikonomou E, Foros P, Tagkli A, Rahiotis C, Eliades T, Koletsi D. Impact of aligners and fixed appliances on oral health during orthodontic treatment: a systematic review and meta-analysis. Oral Health Prev Dent. 2021;19(1):659–72.

23. Ali Baeshen H, El-Bialy T, Alshehri A, Awadh W, Thomas J, Dhillon H, et al. The effect of clear aligners on speech: a systematic review. Eur J Orthod. 2023;45(1):11–9.

24. Nucera R, Dolci C, Bellocchio AM, Costa S, Barbera S, Rustico L, et al. Effects of composite attachments on orthodontic clear aligners therapy: a systematic review. Materials (Basel). 2022;15(2):533.

25. Yassir YA, Nabbat SA, McIntyre GT, Bearn DR. Clinical effectiveness of clear aligner treatment compared to fixed appliance treatment: an overview of systematic reviews. Clin Oral Investig. 2022;26(3):2353–70.

26. Iliadi A, Koletsi D, Eliades T. Forces and moments generated by aligner-type appliances for orthodontic tooth movement: a systematic review and meta-analysis. Orthod Craniofac Res. 2019;22(4):248–58.

27. Schuster S, Eliades G, Zinelis S, Eliades T, Bradley TG. Structural conformation and leaching from in vitro aged and retrieved Invisalign appliances. Am J Orthod Dentofacial Orthop. 2004;126(6):725–8.

28. Gracco A, Mazzoli A, Favoni O, Conti C, Ferraris P, Tosi G, et al. Short-term chemical and physical changes in invisalign appliances. Aust Orthod J. 2009;25(1):34–40.

29. Ryu JH, Kwon JS, Jiang HB, Cha JY, Kim KM. Effects of thermoforming on the physical and mechanical properties of thermoplastic materials for transparent orthodontic aligners. Korean J Orthod. 2018;48(5):316–25.

30. Bucci R, Rongo R, Levate C, Michelotti A, Barone S, Razionale AV, et al. Thickness of orthodontic clear aligners after thermoforming and after 10 days of intraoral exposure: a prospective clinical study. Prog Orthod. 2019;20(1):36.
31. Levrini L, Mangano A, Montanari P, Margherini S, Caprioglio A, Abbate GM. Periodontal health status in patients treated with the Invisalign((R)) system and fixed orthodontic appliances: a 3 months clinical and microbiological evaluation. Eur J Dent. 2015;9(3):404–10.
32. van Gastel J, Quirynen M, Teughels W, Coucke W, Carels C. Longitudinal changes in microbiology and clinical periodontal variables after placement of fixed orthodontic appliances. J Periodontol. 2008;79(11):2078–86.
33. Atack NE, Sandy JR, Addy M. Periodontal and microbiological changes associated with the placement of orthodontic appliances. A review. J Periodontol. 1996;67(2):78–85.
34. Petti S, Barbato E, Simonetti D'Arca A. Effect of orthodontic therapy with fixed and removable appliances on oral microbiota: a six-month longitudinal study. New Microbiol. 1997;20(1):55–62.
35. Gomes SC, Varela CC, da Veiga SL, Rosing CK, Oppermann RV. Periodontal conditions in subjects following orthodontic therapy. A preliminary study. Eur J Orthod. 2007;29(5):477–81.
36. Han JY. A comparative study of combined periodontal and orthodontic treatment with fixed appliances and clear aligners in patients with periodontitis. J Periodontal Implant Sci. 2015;45(6):193–204.
37. Karkhanechi M, Chow D, Sipkin J, Sherman D, Boylan RJ, Norman RG, et al. Periodontal status of adult patients treated with fixed buccal appliances and removable aligners over one year of active orthodontic therapy. Angle Orthod. 2013;83(1):146–51.
38. Turkoz C, Canigur Bavbek N, Kale Varlik S, Akca G. Influence of thermoplastic retainers on Streptococcus mutans and lactobacillus adhesion. Am J Orthod Dentofacial Orthop. 2012;141(5):598–603.
39. Barreda GJ, Dzierewianko EA, Mazza V, Munoz KA, Piccoli GI, Romanelli HJ. Expansion treatment using Invisalign(R): periodontal health status and maxillary buccal bone changes. A clinical and tomographic evaluation. Acta Odontol Latinoam. 2020;33(2):69–81.
40. Dasy H, Dasy A, Asatrian G, Rozsa N, Lee HF, Kwak JH. Effects of variable attachment shapes and aligner material on aligner retention. Angle Orthod. 2015;85(6):934–40.
41. Simon M, Keilig L, Schwarze J, Jung BA, Bourauel C. Treatment outcome and efficacy of an aligner technique—regarding incisor torque, premolar derotation and molar distalization. BMC Oral Health. 2014;14:68.
42. Krieger E, Seiferth J, Marinello I, Jung BA, Wriedt S, Jacobs C, et al. Invisalign(R) treatment in the anterior region: were the predicted tooth movements achieved? J Orofac Orthop. 2012;73(5):365–76.
43. Li W, Wang S, Zhang Y. The effectiveness of the Invisalign appliance in extraction cases using the ABO model grading system: a multicenter randomized controlled trial. Int J Clin Exp Med. 2015;8(5):8276–82.
44. Kassam SK, Stoops FR. Are clear aligners as effective as conventional fixed appliances? Evid Based Dent. 2020;21(1):30–1.
45. D'Anto V, Bucci R, De Simone V, Huanca Ghislanzoni L, Michelotti A, Rongo R. Evaluation of tooth movement accuracy with aligners: a prospective study. Materials (Basel). 2022;15(7):2646.
46. Joffe L. Invisalign: early experiences. J Orthod. 2003;30(4):348–52.
47. Kravitz ND, Kusnoto B, BeGole E, Obrez A, Agran B. How well does Invisalign work? A prospective clinical study evaluating the efficacy of tooth movement with Invisalign. Am J Orthod Dentofacial Orthop. 2009;135(1):27–35.
48. Gu J, Tang JS, Skulski B, Fields HW Jr, Beck FM, Firestone AR, et al. Evaluation of Invisalign treatment effectiveness and efficiency compared with conventional fixed appliances using the peer assessment rating index. Am J Orthod Dentofacial Orthop. 2017;151(2):259–66.
49. Djeu G, Shelton C, Maganzini A. Outcome assessment of Invisalign and traditional orthodontic treatment compared with the American Board of Orthodontics objective grading system. Am J Orthod Dentofacial Orthop. 2005;128(3):292–8. discussion 8.

50. Zhang XJ, He L, Guo HM, Tian J, Bai YX, Li S. Integrated three-dimensional digital assessment of accuracy of anterior tooth movement using clear aligners. Korean J Orthod. 2015;45(6):275–81.
51. Pavoni C, Lione R, Lagana G, Cozza P. Self-ligating versus Invisalign: analysis of dento-alveolar effects. Ann Stomatol (Roma). 2011;2(1–2):23–7.
52. Kuncio D, Maganzini A, Shelton C, Freeman K. Invisalign and traditional orthodontic treatment postretention outcomes compared using the American Board of Orthodontics objective grading system. Angle Orthod. 2007;77(5):864–9.
53. Timm LH, Farrag G, Baxmann M, Schwendicke F. Factors influencing patient compliance during clear aligner therapy: a retrospective cohort study. J Clin Med. 2021;10(14):3103.
54. Bilello G, Fazio M, Amato E, Crivello L, Galvano A, Curro G. Accuracy evaluation of orthodontic movements with aligners: a prospective observational study. Prog Orthod. 2022;23(1):12.
55. Christou T, Betlej A, Aswad N, Ogdon D, Kau CH. Clinical effectiveness of orthodontic treatment on smile esthetics: a systematic review. Clin Cosmet Investig Dent. 2019;11:89–101.
56. Jiang T, Jiang YN, Chu FT, Lu PJ, Tang GH. A cone-beam computed tomographic study evaluating the efficacy of incisor movement with clear aligners: assessment of incisor pure tipping, controlled tipping, translation, and torque. Am J Orthod Dentofacial Orthop. 2021;159(5):635–43.
57. Al-Balaa M, Li H, Ma Mohamed A, Xia L, Liu W, Chen Y, et al. Predicted and actual outcome of anterior intrusion with Invisalign assessed with cone-beam computed tomography. Am J Orthod Dentofacial Orthop. 2021;159(3):e275–e80.
58. Rask H, English JD, Colville C, Kasper FK, Gallerano R, Jacob HB. Cephalometric evaluation of changes in vertical dimension and molar position in adult non-extraction treatment with clear aligners and traditional fixed appliances. Dental Press J Orthod. 2021;26(4):e2119360.
59. Wu D, Zhao Y, Ma M, Zhang Q, Lei H, Wang Y, et al. Efficacy of mandibular molar distalization by clear aligner treatment. Zhong Nan Da Xue Xue Bao Yi Xue Ban. 2021;46(10):1114–21.
60. Yi J, Xiao J, Li Y, Li X, Zhao Z. External apical root resorption in non-extraction cases after clear aligner therapy or fixed orthodontic treatment. J Dent Sci. 2018;13(1):48–53.
61. Eissa O, Carlyle T, El-Bialy T. Evaluation of root length following treatment with clear aligners and two different fixed orthodontic appliances. A pilot study. J Orthod Sci. 2018;7:11.
62. Gandhi V, Mehta S, Gauthier M, Mu J, Kuo CL, Nanda R, et al. Comparison of external apical root resorption with clear aligners and pre-adjusted edgewise appliances in non-extraction cases: a systematic review and meta-analysis. Eur J Orthod. 2021;43(1):15–24.
63. Jyotirmay SSK, Adarsh K, Kumar A, Gupta AR, Sinha A. Comparison of apical root resorption in patients treated with fixed orthodontic appliance and clear aligners: a cone-beam computed tomography study. J Contemp Dent Pract. 2021;22(7):763–8.
64. Liu W, Shao J, Li S, Al-Balaa M, Xia L, Li H, et al. Volumetric cone-beam computed tomography evaluation and risk factor analysis of external apical root resorption with clear aligner therapy. Angle Orthod. 2021;91(5):597–603.
65. Toyokawa-Sperandio KC, Conti A, Fernandes TMF, Almeida-Pedrin RR, Almeida MR, Oltramari PVP. External apical root resorption 6 months after initiation of orthodontic treatment: a randomized clinical trial comparing fixed appliances and orthodontic aligners. Korean J Orthod. 2021;51(5):329–36.
66. Lundstrom F, Krasse B. Streptococcus mutans and lactobacilli frequency in orthodontic patients; the effect of chlorhexidine treatments. Eur J Orthod. 1987;9(2):109–16.
67. Lundstrom F, Krasse B. Caries incidence in orthodontic patients with high levels of streptococcus mutans. Eur J Orthod. 1987;9(2):117–21.
68. Sifakakis I, Papaioannou W, Papadimitriou A, Kloukos D, Papageorgiou SN, Eliades T. Salivary levels of cariogenic bacterial species during orthodontic treatment with thermoplastic aligners or fixed appliances: a prospective cohort study. Prog Orthod. 2018;19(1):25.
69. Zhao R, Huang R, Long H, Li Y, Gao M, Lai W. The dynamics of the oral microbiome and oral health among patients receiving clear aligner orthodontic treatment. Oral Dis. 2020;26(2):473–83.

70. Mummolo S, Tieri M, Nota A, Caruso S, Darvizeh A, Albani F, et al. Salivary concentrations of Streptococcus mutans and Lactobacilli during an orthodontic treatment. An observational study comparing fixed and removable orthodontic appliances. Clin Exp Dent Res. 2020;6(2):181–7.

71. Contaldo M, Lucchese A, Lajolo C, Rupe C, Di Stasio D, Romano A, et al. The oral microbiota changes in orthodontic patients and effects on oral health: an overview. J Clin Med. 2021;10(4):780.

72. Lombardo L, Palone M, Scapoli L, Siciliani G, Carinci F. Short-term variation in the subgingival microbiota in two groups of patients treated with clear aligners and vestibular fixed appliances: a longitudinal study. Orthod Craniofac Res. 2021;24(2):251–60.

73. Shokeen B, Viloria E, Duong E, Rizvi M, Murillo G, Mullen J, et al. The impact of fixed orthodontic appliances and clear aligners on the oral microbiome and the association with clinical parameters: a longitudinal comparative study. Am J Orthod Dentofacial Orthop. 2022;161(5):e475–e85.

74. Kankam H, Madari S, Sawh-Martinez R, Bruckman KC, Steinbacher DM. Comparing outcomes in orthognathic surgery using clear aligners versus conventional fixed appliances. J Craniofac Surg. 2019;30(5):1488–91.

75. Kook MS, Kim HM, Oh HK, Lee KM. Clear aligner use following surgery-first mandibular prognathism correction. J Craniofac Surg. 2019;30(6):e544–e7.

76. Zhang W, Yang H. Orthognathic surgery in Invisalign patients. J Craniofac Surg. 2022;33(2):e112–e3.

77. Aziz SB, Singh G. Cytokine levels in gingival crevicular fluid samples of patients wearing clear aligners. J Oral Biol Craniofac Res. 2020;10(2):199–202.

78. Nota A, Caruso S, Ehsani S, Ferrazzano GF, Gatto R, Tecco S. Short-term effect of orthodontic treatment with clear aligners on pain and sEMG activity of masticatory muscles. Medicina (Kaunas). 2021;57(2):178.

79. AlSeraidi M, Hansa I, Dhaval F, Ferguson DJ, Vaid NR. The effect of vestibular, lingual, and aligner appliances on the quality of life of adult patients during the initial stages of orthodontic treatment. Prog Orthod. 2021;22(1):3.

80. Gao M, Yan X, Zhao R, Shan Y, Chen Y, Jian F, et al. Comparison of pain perception, anxiety, and impacts on oral health-related quality of life between patients receiving clear aligners and fixed appliances during the initial stage of orthodontic treatment. Eur J Orthod. 2021;43(3):353–9.

81. Alfawal AMH, Burhan AS, Mahmoud G, Ajaj MA, Nawaya FR, Hanafi I. The impact of non-extraction orthodontic treatment on oral health-related quality of life: clear aligners versus fixed appliances-a randomized controlled trial. Eur J Orthod. 2022;44:595.

82. Jaber ST, Hajeer MY, Burhan AS, Latifeh Y. The effect of treatment with clear aligners versus fixed appliances on Oral health-related quality of life in patients with severe crowding: a one-year follow-up randomized controlled clinical trial. Cureus. 2022;14(5):e25472.

83. Haydar B, Karabulut G, Ozkan S, Aksoy AU, Ciger S. Effects of retainers on the articulation of speech. Am J Orthod Dentofacial Orthop. 1996;110(5):535–40.

84. Wan J, Wang T, Pei X, Wan Q, Feng W, Chen J. Speech effects of Hawley and vacuum-formed retainers by acoustic analysis: a single-center randomized controlled trial. Angle Orthod. 2017;87(2):286–92.

85. Nedwed V, Miethke RR. Motivation, acceptance and problems of invisalign patients. J Orofac Orthop. 2005;66(2):162–73.

86. Pogal-Sussman-Gandia CB, Tabbaa S, Al-Jewair T. Effects of Invisalign((R)) treatment on speech articulation. Int Orthod. 2019;17(3):513–8.

87. Damasceno Melo PE, Bocato JR, de Castro Ferreira Conti AC, Siqueira de Souza KR, Freire Fernandes TM, de Almeida MR, et al. Effects of orthodontic treatment with aligners and fixed appliances on speech. Angle Orthod. 2021;91(6):711–7.

References

1. Tamer I, Oztas E, Marsan G. Orthodontic treatment with clear aligners and the scientific reality behind their marketing: a literature review. Turk J Orthod. 2019;32(4):241–6.
2. Macrì MMG, Varvara G, Traini T, Festa F. Clinical performances and biological features of clear aligners materials in orthodontics. Front Mater. 2022;9:1–10.
3. Bucci R, Rongo R, Levate C, Michelotti A, Barone S, Razionale AV, et al. Thickness of orthodontic clear aligners after thermoforming and after 10 days of intraoral exposure: a prospective clinical study. Prog Orthod. 2019;20(1):36.
4. Miethke RR, Brauner K. A comparison of the periodontal health of patients during treatment with the Invisalign system and with fixed lingual appliances. J Orofac Orthop. 2007;68(3):223–31.
5. White DW, Julien KC, Jacob H, Campbell PM, Buschang PH. Discomfort associated with Invisalign and traditional brackets: a randomized, prospective trial. Angle Orthod. 2017;87(6):801–8.
6. Flores-Mir C, Brandelli J, Pacheco-Pereira C. Patient satisfaction and quality of life status after 2 treatment modalities: Invisalign and conventional fixed appliances. Am J Orthod Dentofacial Orthop. 2018;154(5):639–44.
7. Zhang B, Huang X, Huo S, Zhang C, Zhao S, Cen X, et al. Effect of clear aligners on oral health-related quality of life: a systematic review. Orthod Craniofac Res. 2020;23(4):363–70.
8. Sangalli L, Savoldi F, Dalessandri D, Bonetti S, Gu M, Signoroni A, et al. Effects of remote digital monitoring on oral hygiene of orthodontic patients: a prospective study. BMC Oral Health. 2021;21(1):435.
9. Rossini G, Parrini S, Castroflorio T, Deregibus A, Debernardi CL. Efficacy of clear aligners in controlling orthodontic tooth movement: a systematic review. Angle Orthod. 2015;85(5):881–9.
10. Zheng M, Liu R, Ni Z, Yu Z. Efficiency, effectiveness and treatment stability of clear aligners: a systematic review and meta-analysis. Orthod Craniofac Res. 2017;20(3):127–33.
11. Kankam HKN, Gupta H, Sawh-Martinez R, Steinbacher DM. Segmental multiple-jaw surgery without orthodontia: clear aligners alone. Plast Reconstr Surg. 2018;142(1):181–4.
12. Sycinska-Dziarnowska M, Szyszka-Sommerfeld L, Wozniak K, Lindauer SJ, Spagnuolo G. Predicting interest in orthodontic aligners: a google trends data analysis. Int J Environ Res Public Health. 2022;19(5):3105.
13. Dasy H, Dasy A, Asatrian G, Rozsa N, Lee HF, Kwak JH. Effects of variable attachment shapes and aligner material on aligner retention. Angle Orthod. 2015;85(6):934–40.
14. Lombardo L, Arreghini A, Bratti E, Mollica F, Spedicato G, Merlin M, et al. Comparative analysis of real and ideal wire-slot play in square and rectangular archwires. Angle Orthod. 2015;85(5):848–58.
15. Liu CL, Sun WT, Liao W, Lu WX, Li QW, Jeong Y, et al. Colour stabilities of three types of orthodontic clear aligners exposed to staining agents. Int J Oral Sci. 2016;8(4):246–53.

© The Editor(s) (if applicable) and The Author(s), under exclusive license to Springer Nature Switzerland AG 2024 177
S. Abela, *Aligner Systems in Invisible Orthodontics*,
https://doi.org/10.1007/978-3-031-49204-4

16. Eliades T, Bourauel C. Intraoral aging of orthodontic materials: the picture we miss and its clinical relevance. Am J Orthod Dentofacial Orthop. 2005;127(4):403–12.
17. Alexandropoulos A, Al Jabbari YS, Zinelis S, Eliades T. Chemical and mechanical characteristics of contemporary thermoplastic orthodontic materials. Aust Orthod J. 2015;31(2):165–70.
18. Edelmann A, English JD, Chen SJ, Kasper FK. Analysis of the thickness of 3-dimensional-printed orthodontic aligners. Am J Orthod Dentofacial Orthop. 2020;158(5):e91–e8.
19. Ren C, Li X, Wang Z, Wang H, Bai Y. Measurement of orthodontic forces exerted on the upper right central incisor with the increase of the distance of tooth movement and thickness of the aligner. Zhonghua Kou Qiang Yi Xue Za Zhi. 2014;49(3):177–9.
20. Elshazly TM, Keilig L, Alkabani Y, Ghoneima A, Abuzayda M, Talaat W, Talaat S, Bourauel C. Potential application of 4D technology in fabrication of orthodontic aligners. Front Mater. 2022;8:794536.
21. Vlaskalic V, Boyd R. Orthodontic treatment of a mildly crowded malocclusion using the Invisalign system. Aust Orthod J. 2001;17(1):41–6.
22. Phan X, Ling PH. Clinical limitations of Invisalign. J Can Dent Assoc. 2007;73(3):263–6.
23. Duncan LO, Piedade L, Lekic M, Cunha RS, Wiltshire WA. Changes in mandibular incisor position and arch form resulting from Invisalign correction of the crowded dentition treated nonextraction. Angle Orthod. 2016;86(4):577–83.
24. Baldwin DK, King G, Ramsay DS, Huang G, Bollen AM. Activation time and material stiffness of sequential removable orthodontic appliances. Part 3: premolar extraction patients. Am J Orthod Dentofacial Orthop. 2008;133(6):837–45.
25. Drake CT, McGorray SP, Dolce C, Nair M, Wheeler TT. Orthodontic tooth movement with clear aligners. ISRN Dent. 2012;2012:657973.
26. Jaber ST, Hajeer MY, Burhan AS, Latifeh Y. The effect of treatment with clear aligners versus fixed appliances on Oral health-related quality of life in patients with severe crowding: a one-year follow-up randomized controlled clinical trial. Cureus. 2022;14(5):e25472.
27. Ben Gassem AA. Does clear aligner treatment result in different patient perceptions of treatment process and outcomes compared to conventional/traditional fixed appliance treatment: a literature review. Eur J Dent. 2022;16(2):274–85.
28. Djeu G, Shelton C, Maganzini A. Outcome assessment of Invisalign and traditional orthodontic treatment compared with the American Board of Orthodontics objective grading system. Am J Orthod Dentofacial Orthop. 2005;128(3):292–8. discussion 8.
29. Kravitz ND, Kusnoto B, BeGole E, Obrez A, Agran B. How well does Invisalign work? A prospective clinical study evaluating the efficacy of tooth movement with Invisalign. Am J Orthod Dentofacial Orthop. 2009;135(1):27–35.
30. Li W, Wang S, Zhang Y. The effectiveness of the Invisalign appliance in extraction cases using the ABO model grading system: a multicenter randomized controlled trial. Int J Clin Exp Med. 2015;8(5):8276–82.
31. Jaber ST, Hajeer MY, Burhan AS. The effectiveness of in-house clear aligners and traditional fixed appliances in achieving good occlusion in complex orthodontic cases: a randomized control clinical trial. Cureus. 2022;14(10):e30147.
32. Nguyen TT, Jackson TH. 3D technologies for precision in orthodontics. Semin Orthod. 2018;24:386.
33. Deferm JT, Schreurs R, Baan F, Bruggink R, Merkx MAW, Xi T, et al. Validation of 3D documentation of palatal soft tissue shape, color, and irregularity with intraoral scanning. Clin Oral Investig. 2018;22(3):1303–9.
34. Isaacson K, Thom AR. Orthodontic radiography guidelines. Am J Orthod Dentofacial Orthop. 2015;147(3):295–6.
35. Condo R, Pazzini L, Cerroni L, Pasquantonio G, Lagana G, Pecora A, et al. Mechanical properties of "two generations" of teeth aligners: change analysis during oral permanence. Dent Mater J. 2018;37(5):835–42.
36. Condo R, Mampieri G, Giancotti A, Cerroni L, Pasquantonio G, Divizia A, et al. SEM characterization and ageing analysis on two generation of invisible aligners. BMC Oral Health. 2021;21(1):316.

37. Bakdach WMM, Haiba M, Hadad R. Changes in surface morphology, chemical and mechanical properties of clear aligners during intraoral usage: a systematic review and meta-analysis. Int Orthod. 2022;20(1):100610.

38. Bruno GGA, Barone M, Mutinelli S, De Stefani A. Invisalign® vs. SparkTM template: which is the most effective in the attachment bonding procedure? A randomized controlled trial. Appl Sci. 2021;11(15):1–6.

39. Mantovani E, Castroflorio E, Rossini G, Garino F, Cugliari G, Deregibus A, et al. Scanning electron microscopy analysis of aligner fitting on anchorage attachments. J Orofac Orthop. 2019;80(2):79–87.

40. Mantovani E, Castroflorio E, Rossini G, Garino F, Cugliari G, Deregibus A, et al. Scanning electron microscopy evaluation of aligner fit on teeth. Angle Orthod. 2018;88(5):596–601.

41. Lombardo L, Palone M, Longo M, Arveda N, Nacucchi M, De Pascalis F, et al. MicroCT X-ray comparison of aligner gap and thickness of six brands of aligners: an in-vitro study. Prog Orthod. 2020;21(1):12.

42. Ryokawa H, Miyazaki Y, Fujishima A, Miyazaki T, Maki K. The mechanical properties of dental thermoplastic materials in a simulated intraoral environment. Orthod Waves. 2006;65(2):64–72.

43. Lombardo L, Martines E, Mazzanti V, Arreghini A, Mollica F, Siciliani G. Stress relaxation properties of four orthodontic aligner materials: a 24-hour in vitro study. Angle Orthod. 2017;87(1):11–8.

44. Palone M, Longo M, Arveda N, Nacucchi M, Pascalis F, Spedicato GA, et al. Micro-computed tomography evaluation of general trends in aligner thickness and gap width after thermoforming procedures involving six commercial clear aligners: an in vitro study. Korean J Orthod. 2021;51(2):135–41.

45. Haouili N, Kravitz ND, Vaid NR, Ferguson DJ, Makki L. Has Invisalign improved? A prospective follow-up study on the efficacy of tooth movement with Invisalign. Am J Orthod Dentofacial Orthop. 2020;158(3):420–5.

46. Sachdev S, Tantidhnazet S, Saengfai NN. Accuracy of tooth movement with in-house clear aligners. J World Fed Orthod. 2021;10(4):177–82.

47. Upadhyay M, Arqub SA. Biomechanics of clear aligners: hidden truths & first principles. J World Fed Orthod. 2022;11(1):12–21.

48. British Standards Institute. Glossary of dental terms (BS 4492). London: BSI; 1983.

49. Karras T, Singh M, Karkazis E, Liu D, Nimeri G, Ahuja B. Efficacy of Invisalign attachments: a retrospective study. Am J Orthod Dentofacial Orthop. 2021;160(2):250–8.

50. Ho CT, Huang YT, Chao CW, Huang TH, Kao CT. Effects of different aligner materials and attachments on orthodontic behavior. J Dent Sci. 2021;16(3):1001–9.

51. Yaosen C, Mohamed AM, Jinbo W, Ziwei Z, Al-Balaa M, Yan Y. Risk factors of composite attachment loss in orthodontic patients during orthodontic clear aligner therapy: a prospective study. Biomed Res Int. 2021;2021:6620377.

52. Bolton WA. Disharmony in tooth size and its relation to the analysis and treatment of malocclusion*. Angle Orthod. 1958;28(3):113–30.

53. Lapenaite E, Lopatiene K. Interproximal enamel reduction as a part of orthodontic treatment. Stomatologija. 2014;16(1):19–24.

54. Stroud JL, English J, Buschang PH. Enamel thickness of the posterior dentition: its implications for nonextraction treatment. Angle Orthod. 1998;68(2):141–6.

55. Tarnow DP, Magner AW, Fletcher P. The effect of the distance from the contact point to the crest of bone on the presence or absence of the interproximal dental papilla. J Periodontol. 1992;63(12):995–6.

56. Meredith L, Mei L, Cannon RD, Farella M. Interproximal reduction in orthodontics: why, where, how much to remove? Aust Orthod J. 2017;33(2):150–7.

57. Peck H, Peck S. An index for assessing tooth shape deviations as applied to the mandibular incisors. Am J Orthod. 1972;61(4):384–401.

58. Gilmore CA, Little RM. Mandibular incisor dimensions and crowding. Am J Orthod. 1984;86(6):493–502.

59. Boese LR. Fiberotomy and reproximation without lower retention, nine years in retrospect: part I. Angle Orthod. 1980;50(2):88–97.

60. Boese LR. Fiberotomy and reproximation without lower retention 9 years in retrospect: part II. Angle Orthod. 1980;50(3):169–78.

61. Kalemaj Z, Levrini L. Quantitative evaluation of implemented interproximal enamel reduction during aligner therapy. Angle Orthod. 2021;91(1):61–6.

62. Jarjoura K, Gagnon G, Nieberg L. Caries risk after interproximal enamel reduction. Am J Orthod Dentofacial Orthop. 2006;130(1):26–30.

63. Kailasam V, Rangarajan H, Easwaran HN, Muthu MS. Proximal enamel thickness of the permanent teeth: a systematic review and meta-analysis. Am J Orthod Dentofacial Orthop. 2021;160(6):793–804 e3.

64. Sarig R, Vardimon AD, Sussan C, Benny L, Sarne O, Hershkovitz I, et al. Pattern of maxillary and mandibular proximal enamel thickness at the contact area of the permanent dentition from first molar to first molar. Am J Orthod Dentofacial Orthop. 2015;147(4):435–44.

65. Zhou N, Guo J. Efficiency of upper arch expansion with the Invisalign system. Angle Orthod. 2020;90(1):23–30.

66. Lione R, Paoloni V, Bartolommei L, Gazzani F, Meuli S, Pavoni C, et al. Maxillary arch development with Invisalign system. Angle Orthod. 2021;91(4):433–40.

67. Levrini L, Carganico A, Abbate L. Maxillary expansion with clear aligners in the mixed dentition: a preliminary study with Invisalign(R) first system. Eur J Paediatr Dent. 2021;22(2):125–8.

68. Ravera S, Castroflorio T, Garino F, Daher S, Cugliari G, Deregibus A. Maxillary molar distalization with aligners in adult patients: a multicenter retrospective study. Prog Orthod. 2016;17:12.

69. Lombardo L, Colonna A, Carlucci A, Oliverio T, Siciliani G. Class II subdivision correction with clear aligners using intermaxilary elastics. Prog Orthod. 2018;19(1):32.

70. Patterson BD, Foley PF, Ueno H, Mason SA, Schneider PP, Kim KB. Class II malocclusion correction with Invisalign: is it possible? Am J Orthod Dentofacial Orthop. 2021;159(1): e41–e8.

71. Carriere L. A new class II distalizer. J Clin Orthod. 2004;38(4):224–31.

72. Kim-Berman H, McNamara JA Jr, Lints JP, McMullen C, Franchi L. Treatment effects of the Carriere((R)) motion 3D appliance for the correction of class II malocclusion in adolescents. Angle Orthod. 2019;89(6):839–46.

73. Henick D, Dayan W, Dunford R, Warunek S, Al-Jewair T. Effects of Invisalign (G5) with virtual bite ramps for skeletal deep overbite malocclusion correction in adults. Angle Orthod. 2021;91(2):164–70.

74. Alsheikho HO, Jomah D. A simple technique to fabricate bite turbos. J Indian Orthod Soc. 2021;55(3):331–5.

75. Vibhute PJ, Srivastava S, Hazarey PV. Temporary bite-raising crowns. J Clin Orthod. 2006;40(4):224–30. quiz 31

76. Roy AS, Singh GK, Tandon P, De N. An interim bite raiser. Int J Orthod Milwaukee. 2013;24(2):63–4.

77. Kravitz ND, Jorgensen G, Frey S, Cope J. Resin bite turbos. J Clin Orthod. 2018;52(9):456–61.

78. Al-Zoubi EM, Al-Nimri KS. A comparative study between the effect of reverse curve of Spee archwires and anterior bite turbos in the treatment of deep overbite cases. Angle Orthod. 2022;92(1):36–44.

79. Khosravi R, Cohanim B, Hujoel P, Daher S, Neal M, Liu W, et al. Management of overbite with the Invisalign appliance. Am J Orthod Dentofacial Orthop. 2017;151(4):691–9 e2.

80. Al-Balaa M, Li H, Ma Mohamed A, Xia L, Liu W, Chen Y, et al. Predicted and actual outcome of anterior intrusion with Invisalign assessed with cone-beam computed tomography. Am J Orthod Dentofacial Orthop. 2021;159(3):e275–e80.

81. Ng J, Major PW, Heo G, Flores-Mir C. True incisor intrusion attained during orthodontic treatment: a systematic review and meta-analysis. Am J Orthod Dentofacial Orthop. 2005;128(2):212–9.

82. Ng J, Major PW, Flores-Mir C. True molar intrusion attained during orthodontic treatment: a systematic review. Am J Orthod Dentofacial Orthop. 2006;130(6):709–14.

83. Greco M, Rombola A. Precision bite ramps and aligners: an elective choice for deep bite treatment. J Orthod. 2022;49(2):213–20.

84. Ng CS, Wong WK, Hagg U. Orthodontic treatment of anterior open bite. Int J Paediatr Dent. 2008;18(2):78–83.

85. Avrella MT, Zimmermann DR, Andriani JSP, Santos PS, Barasuol JC. Prevalence of anterior open bite in children and adolescents: a systematic review and meta-analysis. Eur Arch Paediatr Dent. 2022;23(3):355–64.

86. Moshiri S, Araujo EA, McCray JF, Thiesen G, Kim KB. Cephalometric evaluation of adult anterior open bite non-extraction treatment with Invisalign. Dental Press J Orthod. 2017;22(5):30–8.

87. Kim K, Choy K, Park YC, Han SY, Jung H, Choi YJ. Prediction of mandibular movement and its center of rotation for nonsurgical correction of anterior open bite via maxillary molar intrusion. Angle Orthod. 2018;88(5):538–44.

88. Abuzinada S, Alsulaimani F. Mandibular changes associated with maxillary impaction and molar intrusion. Open J Stomatol. 2013;3:515–9.

89. Park YC, Lee SY, Kim DH, Jee SH. Intrusion of posterior teeth using mini-screw implants. Am J Orthod Dentofacial Orthop. 2003;123(6):690–4.

90. Talens-Cogollos L, Vela-Hernandez A, Peiro-Guijarro MA, Garcia-Sanz V, Montiel-Company JM, Gandia-Franco JL, et al. Unplanned molar intrusion after Invisalign treatment. Am J Orthod Dentofacial Orthop. 2022;162(4):451–8.

91. Destang DL, Kerr WJ. Maxillary retention: is longer better? Eur J Orthod. 2003;25(1):65–9.

92. Littlewood SJ, Mitchell L. An introduction to orthodontics. Oxford university Press; 2019.

93. Pithon MM. A modified thermoplastic retainer. Prog Orthod. 2012;13(2):195–9.

94. Ragunanthanan LMU, Vijayalakshmi D. Comparison of settling of occlusion in modified and full coverage thermoplastic retainers using T-scan. APOS Trends Orthod. 2022;12:115–24.

95. Sari Z, Uysal T, Basciftci FA, Inan O. Occlusal contact changes with removable and bonded retainers in a 1-year retention period. Angle Orthod. 2009;79(5):867–72.

96. Adkins MD, Nanda RS, Currier GF. Arch perimeter changes on rapid palatal expansion. Am J Orthod Dentofacial Orthop. 1990;97(3):194–9.

97. Wertz RA. Skeletal and dental changes accompanying rapid midpalatal suture opening. Am J Orthod. 1970;58(1):41–66.

98. Lopez-Gavito G, Wallen TR, Little RM, Joondeph DR. Anterior open-bite malocclusion: a longitudinal 10-year postretention evaluation of orthodontically treated patients. Am J Orthod. 1985;87(3):175–86.

99. Greenlee GM, Huang GJ, Chen SS, Chen J, Koepsell T, Hujoel P. Stability of treatment for anterior open-bite malocclusion: a meta-analysis. Am J Orthod Dentofacial Orthop. 2011;139(2):154–69.

100. Salehi P, Pakshir HR, Hoseini SA. Evaluating the stability of open bite treatments and its predictive factors in the retention phase during permanent dentition. J Dent (Shiraz). 2015;16(1):22–9.

101. Janson G, Valarelli FP, Henriques JF, de Freitas MR, Cancado RH. Stability of anterior open bite nonextraction treatment in the permanent dentition. Am J Orthod Dentofacial Orthop. 2003;124(3):265–76. quiz 340

102. Tanimoto K, Suzuki A, Nakatani Y, Yanagida T, Tanne Y, Tanaka E, et al. A case of anterior open bite with severely narrowed maxillary dental arch and hypertrophic palatine tonsils. J Orthod. 2008;35(1):5–15.

103. Farret MM, Farret MM, Farret AM. Skeletal class III and anterior open bite treatment with different retention protocols: a report of three cases. J Orthod. 2012;39(3):212–23.

104. Albaker BRB, Wong R. A new skeletal retention system for retaining anterior open bites. APOS Trends Orthod. 2013;3:49–53.

105. Sabouni W, Hansa I, Al Ali SM, Adel SM, Vaid N. Invisalign treatment with mandibular advancement: a retrospective cohort cephalometric appraisal. J Clin Imaging Sci. 2022;12:42.

106. Ravera S, Castroflorio T, Galati F, Cugliari G, Garino F, Deregibus A, et al. Short term dentoskeletal effects of mandibular advancement clear aligners in class II growing patients. A prospective controlled study according to STROBE guidelines. Eur J Paediatr Dent. 2021;22(2):119–24.

107. Rongo R, Dianiskova S, Spiezia A, Bucci R, Michelotti A, D'Anto V. Class II malocclusion in adult patients: what are the effects of the Intermaxillary elastics with clear aligners? A retrospective single center one-group longitudinal study. J Clin Med. 2022;11(24):7333.

108. Koukou M, Damanakis G, Tsolakis AI. Orthodontic management of skeletal class II malocclusion with the Invisalign mandibular advancement feature appliance: a case report and review of the literature. Case Rep Dent. 2022;2022:7095467.

109. Theroux KL. A new vacuum-formed phase I retainer. J Clin Orthod. 2003;37(7):384–7.

110. Larsen MK. Indications for orthognathic surgery—A review. Oral Health Dent Manag. 2017;2017:1–13.

111. Cremona M, Bister D, Sheriff M, Abela S. Quality-of-life improvement, psychosocial benefits, and patient satisfaction of patients undergoing orthognathic surgery: a summary of systematic reviews. Eur J Orthod. 2022;44(6):603–13.

112. Marcuzzi E, Galassini G, Procopio O, Castaldo A, Contardo L. Surgical-Invisalign treatment of a patient with class III malocclusion and multiple missing teeth. J Clin Orthod. 2010;44(6):377–84.

113. Pagani R, Signorino F, Poli PP, Manzini P, Panisi I. The use of Invisalign(R) system in the management of the orthodontic treatment before and after class III surgical approach. Case Rep Dent. 2016;2016:9231219.

114. Womack WR, Day RH. Surgical-orthodontic treatment using the Invisalign system. J Clin Orthod. 2008;42(4):237–45.

115. Zhang W, Yang H. Orthognathic surgery in Invisalign patients. J Craniofac Surg. 2022;33(2):e112–e3.

116. Miranda SL, Oliveira MR, Cheim Junior AP, Moreno R, Miranda MVF, Barbosa RLL. Clear aligners combined with orthognathic surgery: a case series. Gen Dent. 2023;71(1):66–70.

117. Kankam H, Madari S, Sawh-Martinez R, Bruckman KC, Steinbacher DM. Comparing outcomes in orthognathic surgery using clear aligners versus conventional fixed appliances. J Craniofac Surg. 2019;30(5):1488–91.

118. Cong A, Ruellas ACO, Tai SK, Loh CT, Barkley M, Yatabe M, et al. Presurgical orthodontic decompensation with clear aligners. Am J Orthod Dentofacial Orthop. 2022;162(4):538–53.

119. Bishara SE. Textbook of orthodontics. Elsevier (A Division of Reed Elsevier India Pvt. Limited); 2001.

120. Houle JP, Piedade L, Todescan R Jr, Pinheiro FH. The predictability of transverse changes with Invisalign. Angle Orthod. 2017;87(1):19–24.

121. Morales-Burruezo I, Gandia-Franco JL, Cobo J, Vela-Hernandez A, Bellot-Arcis C. Arch expansion with the Invisalign system: efficacy and predictability. PLoS One. 2020;15(12):e0242979.

122. Simon M, Keilig L, Schwarze J, Jung BA, Bourauel C. Treatment outcome and efficacy of an aligner technique—regarding incisor torque, premolar derotation and molar distalization. BMC Oral Health. 2014;14:68.

123. Palone M, Casella S, De Sbrocchi A, Siciliani G, Lombardo L. Space closure by miniscrew-assisted mesialization of an upper third molar and partial vestibular fixed appliance: a case report. Int Orthod. 2022;20(1):100602.

124. Wilmes B, Schwarze J, Vasudavan S, Drescher D. Maxillary space closure using aligners and palatal mini-implants in patients with congenitally missing lateral incisors. J Clin Orthod. 2021;55(1):20–33.

125. Wilmes B, Nienkemper M, Nanda R, Lubberink G, Drescher D. Palatally anchored maxillary molar mesialization using the mesialslider. J Clin Orthod. 2013;47(3):172–9.

126. Auladell A, De La Iglesia F, Quevedo O, Walter A, Puigdollers A. The efficiency of molar distalization using clear aligners and mini-implants: two clinical cases. Int Orthod. 2022;20(1):100604.

127. Saif BS, Pan F, Mou Q, Han M, Bu W, Zhao J, et al. Efficiency evaluation of maxillary molar distalization using Invisalign based on palatal rugae registration. Am J Orthod Dentofacial Orthop. 2022;161(4):e372–e9.

128. D'Anto V, Valletta R, Ferretti R, Bucci R, Kirlis R, Rongo R. Predictability of maxillary molar distalization and derotation with clear aligners: a prospective study. Int J Environ Res Public Health. 2023;20(4):2941.

129. Verma P, George AM. Efficacy of clear aligners in producing molar distalization: systematic review. APOS Trends Orthod. 2022;11:317–24.

130. Sada Garralda VJ. Simultaneous intrusion and distalization using miniscrews in the maxillary tuberosity. J Clin Orthod. 2016;50(10):605–12.

131. Wilmes B, Nienkemper M, Ludwig B, Kau CH, Pauls A, Drescher D. Esthetic class II treatment with the Beneslider and aligners. J Clin Orthod. 2012;46(7):390–8; quiz 437.

132. Wilmes B, Nanda R, Nienkemper M, Ludwig B, Drescher D. Correction of upper-arch asymmetries using the Mesial-Distalslider. J Clin Orthod. 2013;47(11):648–55.

133. Lombardo L, Palone M, Carlucci A, Siciliani G. Clear aligner hybrid approach: a case report. J World Fed Orthod. 2020;9(1):32–43.

134. Kassam SK, Stoops FR. Are clear aligners as effective as conventional fixed appliances? Evid Based Dent. 2020;21(1):30–1.

135. Moon C, Sándor GK, Ko EC, Kim Y-D. Postoperative stability of patients undergoing orthognathic surgery with orthodontic treatment using clear aligners: a preliminary study. Appl Sci. 2021;11(23):11216.

136. Robertson L, Kaur H, Fagundes NCF, Romanyk D, Major P, Flores MC. Effectiveness of clear aligner therapy for orthodontic treatment: a systematic review. Orthod Craniofac Res. 2020;23(2):133–42.

137. Gu J, Tang JS, Skulski B, Fields HW Jr, Beck FM, Firestone AR, et al. Evaluation of Invisalign treatment effectiveness and efficiency compared with conventional fixed appliances using the peer assessment rating index. Am J Orthod Dentofacial Orthop. 2017;151(2):259–66.

138. Smith JM, Weir T, Kaang A, Farella M. Predictability of lower incisor tip using clear aligner therapy. Prog Orthod. 2022;23(1):37.

139. Buschang PH, Ross M, Shaw SG, Crosby D, Campbell PM. Predicted and actual end-of-treatment occlusion produced with aligner therapy. Angle Orthod. 2015;85(5):723–7.

140. Krieger E, Seiferth J, Marinello I, Jung BA, Wriedt S, Jacobs C, et al. Invisalign(R) treatment in the anterior region: were the predicted tooth movements achieved? J Orofac Orthop. 2012;73(5):365–76.

141. Riede U, Wai S, Neururer S, Reistenhofer B, Riede G, Bessei K, et al. Maxillary expansion or contraction and occlusal contact adjustment: effectiveness of current aligner treatment. Clin Oral Investig. 2021;25(7):4671–9.

142. Al-Abdallah M, Hamdan M, Dar-Odeh N. Traditional vs digital communication channels for improving compliance with fixed orthodontic treatment. Angle Orthod. 2021;91(2):227–35.

143. Barbosa IV, Ladewig VM, Almeida-Pedrin RR, Cardoso MA, Santiago Junior JF, Conti A. The association between patient's compliance and age with the bonding failure of orthodontic brackets: a cross-sectional study. Prog Orthod. 2018;19(1):11.

144. Timm LH, Farrag G, Baxmann M, Schwendicke F. Factors influencing patient compliance during clear aligner therapy: a retrospective cohort study. J Clin Med. 2021;10(14):3103.

145. Doruk C, Agar U, Babacan H. The role of the headgear timer in extraoral co-operation. Eur J Orthod. 2004;26(3):289–91.

146. Cureton SL, Regennitter F, Orbell MG. An accurate, inexpensive headgear timer. J Clin Orthod. 1991;25(12):749–54.

147. Tuncay OC, Bowman SJ, Nicozisis JL, Amy BD. Effectiveness of a compliance indicator for clear aligners. J Clin Orthod. 2009;43(4):263–8; quiz 73–4

148. Schott TC, Goz G. Color fading of the blue compliance indicator encapsulated in removable clear Invisalign Teen(R) aligners. Angle Orthod. 2011;81(2):185–91.

149. Brezniak N. The clear plastic appliance: a biomechanical point of view. Angle Orthod. 2008;78(2):381–2.

150. Simon M, Keilig L, Schwarze J, Jung BA, Bourauel C. Forces and moments generated by removable thermoplastic aligners: incisor torque, premolar derotation, and molar distalization. Am J Orthod Dentofacial Orthop. 2014;145(6):728–36.
151. Sandhya V, Arun A, Reddy VP, Mahendra S, Chandrashekar B, Aravind. Biomechanical effects of Torquing on upper central incisor with thermoplastic aligner: a comparative three-dimensional finite element study with and without Auxillaries. J Indian Orthod Soc. 2022;56(1):49–56.
152. Castroflorio T, Garino F, Lazzaro A, Debernardi C. Upper-incisor root control with Invisalign appliances. J Clin Orthod. 2013;47(6):346–51; quiz 87
153. Lima BP, Maio Pinzan-Vercelino CR, Dias LS, Bramante FS, De Jesus Tavarez RR. Correlation between the rotation of the first molars and the severity of class II division 1 malocclusion. Sci World J. 2015;2015:261485.
154. Dahlquist A, Gebauer U, Ingervall B. The effect of a transpalatal arch for the correction of first molar rotation. Eur J Orthod. 1996;18(3):257–67.
155. Vigano CO, da Rocha VE, Junior LRM, Paranhos LR, Ramos AL. Rotation of the upper first molar in class I, II, and III patients. Eur J Dent. 2016;10(1):59–63.
156. Yamunadevi A, Pratibha R, Rajmohan M, Mahendraperumal S, Ganapathy N, Srivandhana R. First molars in permanent dentition and their malformations in various pathologies: a review. J Pharm Bioallied Sci. 2021;13(Suppl 1):S23–30.
157. Bishara SE, Hoppens BJ, Jakobsen JR, Kohout FJ. Changes in the molar relationship between the deciduous and permanent dentitions: a longitudinal study. Am J Orthod Dentofacial Orthop. 1988;93(1):19–28.
158. Lamons FF, Holmes CW III. The problem of the rotated maxillary first permanent molar. Am J Orthod. 1961;47(2):246–72.
159. Braun S, Kusnoto B, Evans CA. The effect of maxillary first molar derotation on arch length. Am J Orthod Dentofacial Orthop. 1997;112(5):538–44.
160. Giuntini V, Baccetti T, Defraia E, Cozza P, Franchi L. Mesial rotation of upper first molars in class II division 1 malocclusion in the mixed dentition: a controlled blind study. Prog Orthod. 2011;12(2):107–13.
161. Zachrisson BU. Important aspects of long-term stability. J Clin Orthod. 1997;31(9):562–83.
162. Garino F, Castroflorio T, Daher S, Ravera S, Rossini G, Cugliari G, et al. Effectiveness of composite attachments in controlling upper-molar movement with aligners. J Clin Orthod. 2016;50(6):341–7.
163. Maree A, Kerr B, Weir T, Freer E. Clinical expression of programmed rotation and uprighting of bilateral winged maxillary central incisors with the Invisalign appliance: a retrospective study. Am J Orthod Dentofacial Orthop. 2022;161(1):74–83.
164. Gaddam R, Freer E, Kerr B, Weir T. Reliability of torque expression by the invisalign appliance: a retrospective study. Aust Orthod J. 2021;37(1):3–13.
165. Blundell HLD, Weir TD, Kerr BD, Freer ED. Predictability of overbite control with the Invisalign appliance. Am J Orthod Dentofacial Orthop. 2021;160(5):725–31.
166. Macena MC, Katz CR, Rosenblatt A. Prevalence of a posterior crossbite and sucking habits in Brazilian children aged 18-59 months. Eur J Orthod. 2009;31(4):357–61.
167. Kisling E. Occlusal interferences in the primary dentition. ASDC J Dent Child. 1981;48(3):181–91.
168. Lindner A, Modeer T. Relation between sucking habits and dental characteristics in pre-schoolchildren with unilateral cross-bite. Scand J Dent Res. 1989;97(3):278–83.
169. Almeida RR, Almeida MR, Oltramari-Navarro PV, Conti AC, Navarro Rde L, Marques HV. Posterior crossbite—treatment and stability. J Appl Oral Sci. 2012;20(2):286–94.
170. Beers AC, Choi W, Pavlovskaia E. Computer-assisted treatment planning and analysis. Orthod Craniofac Res. 2003;6(Suppl 1):117–25.
171. Miller RJ, Kuo E, Choi W. Validation of align technology's treat III digital model superimposition tool and its case application. Orthod Craniofac Res. 2003;6(Suppl 1):143–9.
172. Rossini G, Parrini S, Castroflorio T, Deregibus A, Debernardi CL. Periodontal health during clear aligners treatment: a systematic review. Eur J Orthod. 2015;37(5):539–43.

173. Elhaddaoui R, Qoraich HS, Bahije L, Zaoui F. Orthodontic aligners and root resorption: a systematic review. Int Orthod. 2017;15(1):1–12.

174. Aldeeri A, Alhammad L, Alduham A, Ghassan W, Shafshak S, Fatani E. Association of orthodontic clear aligners with root resorption using three-dimension measurements: a systematic review. J Contemp Dent Pract. 2018;19(12):1558–64.

175. Jiang Q, Li J, Mei L, Du J, Levrini L, Abbate GM, et al. Periodontal health during orthodontic treatment with clear aligners and fixed appliances: a meta-analysis. J Am Dent Assoc. 2018;149(8):712–20 e12.

176. Lu H, Tang H, Zhou T, Kang N. Assessment of the periodontal health status in patients undergoing orthodontic treatment with fixed appliances and Invisalign system: a meta-analysis. Medicine (Baltimore). 2018;97(13):e0248.

177. Papadimitriou A, Mousoulea S, Gkantidis N, Kloukos D. Clinical effectiveness of Invisalign(R) orthodontic treatment: a systematic review. Prog Orthod. 2018;19(1):37.

178. Fang X, Qi R, Liu C. Root resorption in orthodontic treatment with clear aligners: a systematic review and meta-analysis. Orthod Craniofac Res. 2019;22(4):259–69.

179. Galan-Lopez L, Barcia-Gonzalez J, Plasencia E. A systematic review of the accuracy and efficiency of dental movements with Invisalign(R). Korean J Orthod. 2019;49(3):140–9.

180. Ke Y, Zhu Y, Zhu M. A comparison of treatment effectiveness between clear aligner and fixed appliance therapies. BMC Oral Health. 2019;19(1):24.

181. Al-Zainal MH, Anvery S, Al-Jewair T. Clear aligner therapy may not prevent but may decrease the incidence of external root resorption compared to full fixed appliances. J Evid Based Dent Pract. 2020;20(2):101438.

182. Cardoso PC, Espinosa DG, Mecenas P, Flores-Mir C, Normando D. Pain level between clear aligners and fixed appliances: a systematic review. Prog Orthod. 2020;21(1):3.

183. Mheissen S, Khan H, Aldandan M. Limited evidence on differences between fixed appliances and clear aligners regarding pain level. Evid Based Dent. 2020;21(4):144–5.

184. Ghandi K, Pieri B, Dornhorst A, Hussain S. A comparison of validated methods used to assess impaired awareness of hypoglycaemia in type 1 diabetes: an observational study. Diabetes Ther. 2021;12(1):441–51.

185. Oikonomou E, Foros P, Tagkli A, Rahiotis C, Eliades T, Koletsi D. Impact of aligners and fixed appliances on oral health during orthodontic treatment: a systematic review and meta-analysis. Oral Health Prev Dent. 2021;19(1):659–72.

186. Ali Baeshen H, El-Bialy T, Alshehri A, Awadh W, Thomas J, Dhillon H, et al. The effect of clear aligners on speech: a systematic review. Eur J Orthod. 2023;45(1):11–9.

187. Nucera R, Dolci C, Bellocchio AM, Costa S, Barbera S, Rustico L, et al. Effects of composite attachments on orthodontic clear aligners therapy: a systematic review. Materials (Basel). 2022;15(2):533.

188. Yassir YA, Nabbat SA, McIntyre GT, Bearn DR. Clinical effectiveness of clear aligner treatment compared to fixed appliance treatment: an overview of systematic reviews. Clin Oral Investig. 2022;26(3):2353–70.

189. Iliadi A, Koletsi D, Eliades T. Forces and moments generated by aligner-type appliances for orthodontic tooth movement: a systematic review and meta-analysis. Orthod Craniofac Res. 2019;22(4):248–58.

190. Schuster S, Eliades G, Zinelis S, Eliades T, Bradley TG. Structural conformation and leaching from in vitro aged and retrieved Invisalign appliances. Am J Orthod Dentofacial Orthop. 2004;126(6):725–8.

191. Gracco A, Mazzoli A, Favoni O, Conti C, Ferraris P, Tosi G, et al. Short-term chemical and physical changes in invisalign appliances. Aust Orthod J. 2009;25(1):34–40.

192. Ryu JH, Kwon JS, Jiang HB, Cha JY, Kim KM. Effects of thermoforming on the physical and mechanical properties of thermoplastic materials for transparent orthodontic aligners. Korean J Orthod. 2018;48(5):316–25.

193. Levrini L, Mangano A, Montanari P, Margherini S, Caprioglio A, Abbate GM. Periodontal health status in patients treated with the Invisalign((R)) system and fixed orthodontic appliances: a 3 months clinical and microbiological evaluation. Eur J Dent. 2015;9(3):404–10.

194. van Gastel J, Quirynen M, Teughels W, Coucke W, Carels C. Longitudinal changes in microbiology and clinical periodontal variables after placement of fixed orthodontic appliances. J Periodontol. 2008;79(11):2078–86.

195. Atack NE, Sandy JR, Addy M. Periodontal and microbiological changes associated with the placement of orthodontic appliances. A review. J Periodontol. 1996;67(2):78–85.

196. Petti S, Barbato E, Simonetti D'Arca A. Effect of orthodontic therapy with fixed and removable appliances on oral microbiota: a six-month longitudinal study. New Microbiol. 1997;20(1):55–62.

197. Gomes SC, Varela CC, da Veiga SL, Rosing CK, Oppermann RV. Periodontal conditions in subjects following orthodontic therapy. A preliminary study. Eur J Orthod. 2007;29(5):477–81.

198. Han JY. A comparative study of combined periodontal and orthodontic treatment with fixed appliances and clear aligners in patients with periodontitis. J Periodontal Implant Sci. 2015;45(6):193–204.

199. Karkhanechi M, Chow D, Sipkin J, Sherman D, Boylan RJ, Norman RG, et al. Periodontal status of adult patients treated with fixed buccal appliances and removable aligners over one year of active orthodontic therapy. Angle Orthod. 2013;83(1):146–51.

200. Turkoz C, Canigur Bavbek N, Kale Varlik S, Akca G. Influence of thermoplastic retainers on Streptococcus mutans and lactobacillus adhesion. Am J Orthod Dentofacial Orthop. 2012;141(5):598–603.

201. Barreda GJ, Dzierewianko EA, Mazza V, Munoz KA, Piccoli GI, Romanelli HJ. Expansion treatment using Invisalign(R): periodontal health status and maxillary buccal bone changes. A clinical and tomographic evaluation. Acta Odontol Latinoam. 2020;33(2):69–81.

202. D'Anto V, Bucci R, De Simone V, Huanca Ghislanzoni L, Michelotti A, Rongo R. Evaluation of tooth movement accuracy with aligners: a prospective study. Materials (Basel). 2022;15(7):2646.

203. Joffe L. Invisalign: early experiences. J Orthod. 2003;30(4):348–52.

204. Zhang XJ, He L, Guo HM, Tian J, Bai YX, Li S. Integrated three-dimensional digital assessment of accuracy of anterior tooth movement using clear aligners. Korean J Orthod. 2015;45(6):275–81.

205. Pavoni C, Lione R, Lagana G, Cozza P. Self-ligating versus Invisalign: analysis of dentoalveolar effects. Ann Stomatol (Roma). 2011;2(1–2):23–7.

206. Kuncio D, Maganzini A, Shelton C, Freeman K. Invisalign and traditional orthodontic treatment postretention outcomes compared using the American Board of Orthodontics objective grading system. Angle Orthod. 2007;77(5):864–9.

207. Bilello G, Fazio M, Amato E, Crivello L, Galvano A, Curro G. Accuracy evaluation of orthodontic movements with aligners: a prospective observational study. Prog Orthod. 2022;23(1):12.

208. Christou T, Betlej A, Aswad N, Ogdon D, Kau CH. Clinical effectiveness of orthodontic treatment on smile esthetics: a systematic review. Clin Cosmet Investig Dent. 2019;11:89–101.

209. Jiang T, Jiang YN, Chu FT, Lu PJ, Tang GH. A cone-beam computed tomographic study evaluating the efficacy of incisor movement with clear aligners: assessment of incisor pure tipping, controlled tipping, translation, and torque. Am J Orthod Dentofacial Orthop. 2021;159(5):635–43.

210. Rask H, English JD, Colville C, Kasper FK, Gallerano R, Jacob HB. Cephalometric evaluation of changes in vertical dimension and molar position in adult non-extraction treatment with clear aligners and traditional fixed appliances. Dental Press J Orthod. 2021;26(4):e2119360.

211. Wu D, Zhao Y, Ma M, Zhang Q, Lei H, Wang Y, et al. Efficacy of mandibular molar distalization by clear aligner treatment. Zhong Nan Da Xue Xue Bao Yi Xue Ban. 2021;46(10):1114–21.

212. Yi J, Xiao J, Li Y, Li X, Zhao Z. External apical root resorption in non-extraction cases after clear aligner therapy or fixed orthodontic treatment. J Dent Sci. 2018;13(1):48–53.

213. Eissa O, Carlyle T, El-Bialy T. Evaluation of root length following treatment with clear aligners and two different fixed orthodontic appliances. A pilot study. J Orthod Sci. 2018;7:11.

214. Gandhi V, Mehta S, Gauthier M, Mu J, Kuo CL, Nanda R, et al. Comparison of external apical root resorption with clear aligners and pre-adjusted edgewise appliances in non-extraction cases: a systematic review and meta-analysis. Eur J Orthod. 2021;43(1):15–24.
215. Jyotirmay SSK, Adarsh K, Kumar A, Gupta AR, Sinha A. Comparison of apical root resorption in patients treated with fixed orthodontic appliance and clear aligners: a cone-beam computed tomography study. J Contemp Dent Pract. 2021;22(7):763–8.
216. Liu W, Shao J, Li S, Al-Balaa M, Xia L, Li H, et al. Volumetric cone-beam computed tomography evaluation and risk factor analysis of external apical root resorption with clear aligner therapy. Angle Orthod. 2021;91(5):597–603.
217. Toyokawa-Sperandio KC, Conti A, Fernandes TMF, Almeida-Pedrin RR, Almeida MR, Oltramari PVP. External apical root resorption 6 months after initiation of orthodontic treatment: a randomized clinical trial comparing fixed appliances and orthodontic aligners. Korean J Orthod. 2021;51(5):329–36.
218. Lundstrom F, Krasse B. Streptococcus mutans and lactobacilli frequency in orthodontic patients; the effect of chlorhexidine treatments. Eur J Orthod. 1987;9(2):109–16.
219. Lundstrom F, Krasse B. Caries incidence in orthodontic patients with high levels of streptococcus mutans. Eur J Orthod. 1987;9(2):117–21.
220. Sifakakis I, Papaioannou W, Papadimitriou A, Kloukos D, Papageorgiou SN, Eliades T. Salivary levels of cariogenic bacterial species during orthodontic treatment with thermoplastic aligners or fixed appliances: a prospective cohort study. Prog Orthod. 2018;19(1):25.
221. Zhao R, Huang R, Long H, Li Y, Gao M, Lai W. The dynamics of the oral microbiome and oral health among patients receiving clear aligner orthodontic treatment. Oral Dis. 2020;26(2):473–83.
222. Mummolo S, Tieri M, Nota A, Caruso S, Darvizeh A, Albani F, et al. Salivary concentrations of Streptococcus mutans and Lactobacilli during an orthodontic treatment. An observational study comparing fixed and removable orthodontic appliances. Clin Exp Dent Res. 2020;6(2):181–7.
223. Contaldo M, Lucchese A, Lajolo C, Rupe C, Di Stasio D, Romano A, et al. The oral microbiota changes in orthodontic patients and effects on oral health: an overview. J Clin Med. 2021;10(4):780.
224. Lombardo L, Palone M, Scapoli L, Siciliani G, Carinci F. Short-term variation in the subgingival microbiota in two groups of patients treated with clear aligners and vestibular fixed appliances: a longitudinal study. Orthod Craniofac Res. 2021;24(2):251–60.
225. Shokeen B, Viloria E, Duong E, Rizvi M, Murillo G, Mullen J, et al. The impact of fixed orthodontic appliances and clear aligners on the oral microbiome and the association with clinical parameters: a longitudinal comparative study. Am J Orthod Dentofacial Orthop. 2022;161(5):e475–e85.
226. Kook MS, Kim HM, Oh HK, Lee KM. Clear aligner use following surgery-first mandibular prognathism correction. J Craniofac Surg. 2019;30(6):e544–e7.
227. Aziz SB, Singh G. Cytokine levels in gingival crevicular fluid samples of patients wearing clear aligners. J Oral Biol Craniofac Res. 2020;10(2):199–202.
228. Nota A, Caruso S, Ehsani S, Ferrazzano GF, Gatto R, Tecco S. Short-term effect of orthodontic treatment with clear aligners on pain and sEMG activity of masticatory muscles. Medicina (Kaunas). 2021;57(2):178.
229. AlSeraidi M, Hansa I, Dhaval F, Ferguson DJ, Vaid NR. The effect of vestibular, lingual, and aligner appliances on the quality of life of adult patients during the initial stages of orthodontic treatment. Prog Orthod. 2021;22(1):3.
230. Gao M, Yan X, Zhao R, Shan Y, Chen Y, Jian F, et al. Comparison of pain perception, anxiety, and impacts on oral health-related quality of life between patients receiving clear aligners and fixed appliances during the initial stage of orthodontic treatment. Eur J Orthod. 2021;43(3):353–9.
231. Alfawal AMH, Burhan AS, Mahmoud G, Ajaj MA, Nawaya FR, Hanafi I. The impact of non-extraction orthodontic treatment on oral health-related quality of life: clear aligners versus fixed appliances-a randomized controlled trial. Eur J Orthod. 2022;44:595.

232. Haydar B, Karabulut G, Ozkan S, Aksoy AU, Ciger S. Effects of retainers on the articulation of speech. Am J Orthod Dentofacial Orthop. 1996;110(5):535–40.
233. Wan J, Wang T, Pei X, Wan Q, Feng W, Chen J. Speech effects of Hawley and vacuum-formed retainers by acoustic analysis: a single-center randomized controlled trial. Angle Orthod. 2017;87(2):286–92.
234. Nedwed V, Miethke RR. Motivation, acceptance and problems of invisalign patients. J Orofac Orthop. 2005;66(2):162–73.
235. Pogal-Sussman-Gandia CB, Tabbaa S, Al-Jewair T. Effects of Invisalign((R)) treatment on speech articulation. Int Orthod. 2019;17(3):513–8.
236. Damasceno Melo PE, Bocato JR, de Castro Ferreira Conti AC, Siqueira de Souza KR, Freire Fernandes TM, de Almeida MR, et al. Effects of orthodontic treatment with aligners and fixed appliances on speech. Angle Orthod. 2021;91(6):711–7.

Index

© The Editor(s) (if applicable) and The Author(s), under exclusive license to Springer Nature Switzerland AG 2024
S. Abela, *Aligner Systems in Invisible Orthodontics*,
https://doi.org/10.1007/978-3-031-49204-4

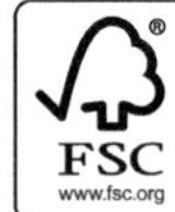